KT-431-725

OXFORD MEDICAL PUBLICATIONS

EATING DISORDERS

the**facts**

WITHDRAWN

Wyggeston QE I

00312207

the**facts**

ALSO PUBLISHED BY OXFORD UNIVERSITY PRESS

EATING DISORDERS

the**facts**

Fifth Edition

By

SUZANNE ABRAHAM
Department of Obstetrics and Gynaecology
University of Sydney
Royal North Shore Hospital

and

DEREK LLEWELLYN-JONES
Previously, *Department of Obstetrics and*
Gynaecology,
University of Sydney

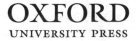

OXFORD
UNIVERSITY PRESS

OXFORD

UNIVERSITY PRESS

Great Clarendon Street, Oxford OX2 6DP

Oxford University Press is a department of the University of Oxford.
It furthers the University's objective of excellence in research, scholarship,
and education by publishing worldwide in

Oxford   New York

Athens   Auckland   Bangkok   Bogotá   Bombay   Buenos Aires   Calcutta
Cape Town   Dar es Salaam   Delhi   Florence   Hong Kong   Istanbul
Karachi   Kuala Lumpur   Madrid   Melbourne   Mexico City   Mumbai
Nairobi Paris   São Paulo   Shanghai   Singapore   Taipei   Tokyo   Toronto   Warsaw

and associated companies in Berlin, Ibadan

Oxford is a registered trade mark of Oxford University Press
in the UK and in certain other countries

Acc. No.

00312207

Class No.

616.8526ABR

Published in the United States
© by Oxford University Press Inc., New York

First edition 1984
Second edition 1987
Third edition 1992
Fourth edition 1997
Fifth edition 2001

Suzanne Abraham and Derek Llewellyn-Jones, 1984, 1987, 1992, 1997, 2001

The moral rights of the author have been asserted

Database right Oxford University Press (maker)

All rights reserved. No part of this publication may be reproduced,
stored in a retrieval system, or transmitted, in any form or by any means,
without the prior permission in writing of Oxford University Press,
or as expressly permitted by law, or under terms agreed with the appropriate
reprographics rights organization. Enquiries concerning reproduction
outside the scope of the above should be sent to the Rights Department,
Oxford University Press, at the address above

You must not circulate this book in any other binding or cover
and you must impose this same condition on any acquirer

British Library Cataloguing in Publication Data
Data available

Library of Congress Cataloguing in Publication Data

Abraham, Suzanne.
Eating disorders: the facts/by Suzanne Abraham and
Derek Llewellyn-Jones.–5th ed. p. cm. — (The facts)
Includes bibliographical references and index.
1. Eating disorders. 2. Bulimia. I. Llewellyn-Jones, Derek. II. Title. III. Facts
(Oxford, England)
RC552.E18 A27 2001   616.85'26—dc21   2001034651

ISBN 0 19 850937 5 (Pb)

Printed in Great Britain by Biddles Ltd, Guildford & King's Lynn

Preface and acknowledgements

Wyggeston QEI College Library

This book has been written for patients, their families, and for health professionals, including family doctors. The reason for including these three groups is that sufferers and their families are increasingly asking for more information, and more young people are presenting to general practitioners with disordered eating, some of whom will have an eating disorder.

In this new edition we have included two new chapters: 'Pregnancy and postpartum' and 'The family'. Pregnancy and caring for a new baby can be major challenges for sufferers of eating disorders. The 'facts' as they are currently known are presented and suggestions made, which we hope will be reassuring both to women desiring pregnancy and their doctors. The chapter 'The family' was included to provide insights from the parents of sufferers of anorexia nervosa and bulimia nervosa.

Studies have shown that the earlier an eating disorder is diagnosed and treatment started the better the outcome is likely to be. Additionally, there is a growing tendency to treat patients with an eating disorder in the community, only admitting to hospital those who need in-patient treatment.

The Facts series does not provide chapter references for published papers (although the authors have them on file). Instead the book suggests 'Further reading' where references can be found.

The fifth edition of *Eating disorders—the facts* could not have been written if we had not had discussions with our colleagues and friends. They include Janice Russell, Michael Mira, Jenny O'Dea, Janet Conti, David Blythe, Louise Kefford, Bianca Pettigrew, Catherine Boyd, Alan Taylor, and the staff of the Eating Disorders Unit at the Northside Clinic, Greenwich, New South Wales.

Most of all we thank our patients. Without them there would be no book. We would particularly like to thank those patients who permitted us to use their emails, letters, diaries, or tape recordings (appropriately modified for reasons of privacy) for the case histories and quotations.

Note

Because of the problems of gender in the English language, we have had to decide whether to use 'he' or 'she' when referring to people. We feel that to use 'person' in each instance is distracting. As we treat more women than men, and as more women than men develop eating disorders, we have chosen to use she rather than he in all instances. The reader should not deduce that we have a sexist bias.

In this book a 'binge' refers to an episode of compulsive overeating, not a drinking bout. We have used the term as our patients describe their eating behaviour as binge-eating.

In many countries the metric system of weights and measures is replacing the older 'imperial' system. We have chosen to express weight as follows: kilograms, pounds, and stones and pounds. We have expressed heights in metres and in feet and inches. This should help readers who find difficulty with the metric system.

Sydney S.A.
July 2001 D.L-J.

the**facts**

CONTENTS

The nosology of insanity, the etiology, the symptomatology, pathology, diagnosis, prognosis, the care—how nicely the textbooks classified everything! How accurately they defined the idiot, the cretin, the imbecile, the epileptic, the hysteric, hypochondriac, and neurasthenic. Instead of admitting that little was known about what went on in the human brain, either healthy or sick, the professors stacked up Latin names.

from *The Estate*
Isaac Bashevis Singer

1
Adolescent eating behaviour

If I was going to get a job when I left school, I felt I had to be half a stone lighter. All my friends were dieting but my mother disapproved. She said it was puppy fat which would disappear. I knew it wouldn't, so I had to pretend I was not hungry because I wanted to be slim.

For most of recorded history a woman was seen as desirable when her body was plump due to the deposition of fat on her breasts, hips, thighs, and abdomen. It was fashionable to be fat. The cultural belief that to be fat was to be attractive was due to the uncertainty of food supplies in pre-industrial and early industrial societies, to the irregular occurrence of famines, and to the effects of diseases which eliminated large numbers of farm labourers. A curvaceous female body indicated that the husband (or father) was prudent, efficient, and affluent. It also indicated that the woman was prepared for times of food shortage. Her family would be protected because she had sufficient food stored in her storeroom to meet the shortage, and she herself had sufficient energy, stored in her body in the form of fat, to look after her family.

In the past 75 years, with abundant food supplies and good food distribution in most of the developed nations of the Western world, almost for the first time in history slimness has begun to become fashionable. This is documented in fashion magazines, in *Playboy* centre-folds, and in records of the 'vital statistics' of women winning beauty contests. For the past three decades the public perception has been that a woman is attractive, desirable, and successful when she is slim. Fashion models have become taller and thinner, and have body weights at least 20 per cent less than a woman of similar age and height living in a consumer society. Body shape, except for changes in preferred breast size, did not receive the same attention as body weight until the 1990s. The features needed to become a successful fashion model have become more detailed and emphasize body shape

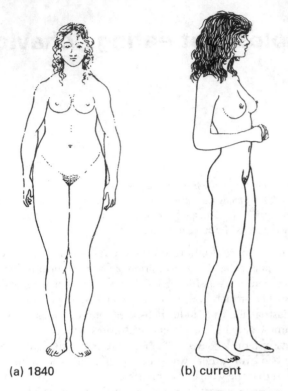

(a) 1840   (b) current

Fig. 1. The changing fashion in women's figures. The first illustration is taken from an obstetrical textbook printed in England in 1840, the second from a current textbook.

in addition to thinness. At the beginning of the twenty-first century the criteria cited by a modelling agency was 'tall, thin, fit but not muscular, brown or tan, strong shouldered, big "well shaped" boobs, small waist, no stomach, small hips, small, high bottom, thin thighs, long legs, and definitely no cellulite or body hair.'

Over the same period, articles on 'new and exciting' diets (often nutritionally inadequate and occasionally dangerous) and exercise programmes have appeared at regular intervals in women's magazines, and the number is increasing. Articles on the problems resulting from cosmetic surgery that promises to produce the perfect body or correct body shape are also increasing.

The media and perception of body shape

Most people living in the developed nations also receive a constant stream of impressions from television commercials which use young, attractive, and slim women to advertise products as diverse as soft drinks, security investments, cars, computers, fast foods, floor polishers etc.

The messages from the media stress how desirable it is for women to be young and to be or to become thin. These messages particularly influence teenage women at a period when they are undergoing emotional stress as they seek to achieve independence from their parents, to compete with their peers, and to find their identity. Adolescence is a time of concern about body image. Achieving the ideal body image is thought to ensure success and happiness.

Hormonal changes in adolescence

In late childhood hormonal changes trigger an increase in height in girls and boys. The increase, or growth spurt, occurs at an earlier age in girls than boys and is achieved by the child increasing the amount of food he or she eats (Fig. 2). In girls the onset of the growth spurt precedes the onset of menstruation and overlaps its

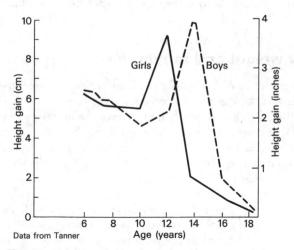

Fig. 2. The 'spurt' in growth at puberty.

establishment at an average age of $12^{1}/_{2}$ years. There is a wide time range in the onset and duration of the growth spurt and the peak may be reached by girls as early as age 10 or as late as age 15 years. The growth spurt is accompanied by marked changes in the bodily appearance of the two sexes, which in turn are dependent on the sex hormones which are now being produced in the girl's ovaries or the boy's testicles. Both sexes show an increase in muscle bulk but this is much more marked in boys. Girls have a particularly large spurt in hip growth resulting in widening of the hips and, in contrast to boys, do not lose fat during the growth spurt. In fact, girls have a general tendency to increase their body fat, particularly on the upper legs, as they cease to gain height. Fat is also deposited beneath the skin, in the breasts and over the hips. Obviously the amount of fat deposited is related to the energy absorbed from the food the girl eats and is influenced by the hormonal changes which are occurring at this time. Energy intake from food is limited by the person's appetite. During early adolescence, unknown factors stimulate the teenager to eat more, with the consequence that the energy intake for girls reaches a maximum during the age range of 11 to 14, at a time when her energy needs are great. From about the age of 14, a teenage girl's energy needs fall, but if she continues to eat the same amount as she has been eating she will absorb an excess of energy which will be converted into fat, and she will become fat. She has to control her food intake, in order to control her weight (Fig. 3).

Body weight and menarche

A clearer picture of the weight challenge young women experience emerges if we look at when women have their first menstrual period rather than their age. Recently we measured the height and weight of over 300 girls aged 11 to 16 and asked them about the weight they would like to be, how they felt about their body appearance, and how many months it had been since their menarche. Body Mass Index (BMI) was calculated from the student's height and weight measures (see page 24) and is shown in Fig. 3. In the 6 to 12 months after a woman has her first period there is a rapid increase in BMI, almost all of which is due to a rapid rise in body weight although women are still growing a small amount in height at this time. The decreasing BMI that occurs more than a year after menarche suggests these students

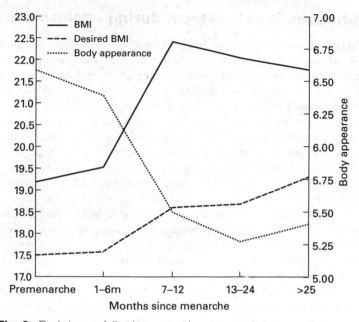

Fig. 3. Body image following menarche.

had changed their eating and exercise habits and lifestyles and were already employing methods of weight loss at this time. The students desired BMI, which is the weight they would like to be for their height, and their rating of their body appearance (out of 10, 10 being best) is also shown (Fig. 3). At all times they wanted their body weight to be less than their actual weight and did not like their body appearance as much after their sudden weight gain in the year after menarche.

This is the adolescent girl's dilemma. She may wish to remain thin or to become thin, because cultural norms expect her to be thin, or she may reject those norms, either because of conflict within herself or within her family, or because she enjoys and finds emotional release in eating. If she chooses to become and remain thin, she has to learn new eating habits, because she will inevitably become fat if she continues eating the quantity of food she has become used to eating and does not increase the amount of exercise she undertakes.

Changes in self-esteem during adolescence

In the early stages of puberty and before menarche most girls feel good about themselves. They feel content with their relationships, their family and friends, their school life, their performance and what they look like. In other words they have a good self-esteem. If you ask them to rate their appearance on a scale from 0 to 10 (10 being best) most rate themselves as 6 or 7. This is the same score adult women give themselves. As a girls growth spurt comes to an end and her first menstrual period occurs she may observe that fat is increasingly being distributed to her breasts, hips, bottom, and thighs. In the 12 months after a woman's first period she is likely to rate her body appearance as 5 or 6 (Fig. 3).

It is these changes around menarche, including weight gain, that are accompanied by a loss of confidence and a decrease in self-esteem among young women. Not only is their opinion of their body appearance poorer but their overall self-esteem is lower; this includes the areas of self-esteem that are valued most by young women; these are, relating well to others and having close relationships, doing well at school or work, and being romantically attractive to others.

Young men are different, their self-esteem increases as they grow taller, become heavier, and increase their muscle mass. In a recent study of pre- and post-pubertal male and female school students we found that post-pubertal male students had the greatest self-esteem and female post-pubertal students the lowest. There was a big discrepancy between what young women feel they 'should be like' and how they 'feel they are'. In other words, young women in their early teens already feel they have failed to reach their expectations of themselves whereas young men were fulfilling their expectations of themselves.

Being overweight and obese in the teenage years also affects students' self-esteem. Overweight (and not obese), young people, both male and female students, have a lower self-esteem than their normal weight male and female peers.

Depression and anxiety during adolescence

Accompanying the changes in self-esteem are changes in other psychological characteristics. A very large epidemiological study found that there is an increase in feelings of depression and anxiety during adolescence for both young men and young women. This change is greatest for young women at the time of their first menstrual period. The results led the researchers to conclude 'menarche marks a transition in the risk for depression and anxiety in young women'. The only other stressful factor found to be associated with depression was divorce of a young woman's parents. The risks for young men are different; these relate to their school year level, the higher the level the greater the risk, and are associated with higher parental expectations of achievement.

One particular type of anxiety called 'social phobia' or 'social anxiety' becomes apparent during puberty. The main feature of social phobia is a fear of embarrassment or humiliation in social situations where the person worries that others are judging their performance. It is a fear of failing in front of others. This can occur when people are eating or speaking in front of other people and in the classroom when someone watches them working. The sufferer may avoid eye contact with people, blush, stop what they are doing, and appear generally anxious. Feeling anxious around people, particularly people they do not know well, is a common worry of people with eating problems.

Perception of 'dieting' around menarche

Until a few months before a woman's first period she usually does not think about dieting and if she is asked the question 'what does dieting mean?' she is likely to describe dieting as 'healthy eating'. It is not until she has grown taller, menstruated, and increased her body weight that her perception of dieting includes the idea that dieting is for loss of body weight. Some pre-pubertal girls, who report dieting for weight loss, are commonly being shown how to diet by their older sister or mother as they wish to avoid becoming like the family members who are overweight or obese. Frequently they 'diet with' their sister or mother and understand dieting is a lifestyle that is to be continued throughout life.

Nine adolescents who were aged 13 years and trying to lose weight were asked the question 'Is dieting different after your first period?'. Their responses are shown in Table 1.

Adolescents' perception of body shape

A young woman's perception of her body is important to her psychological well-being. She may see her body as large and overweight

Table 1. Post-menarchial students trying to lose body weight

After menarche:

- 'dieting becomes more serious and you think about it more'
- 'you start to get more interested (in yourself)'
- 'I put on stacks of weight'
- 'you feel you're getting fat, I don't want to turn out like my step Mum'
- 'after your period you worry about your appearance'
- 'worry what people think – mostly boys'
- 'don't know I've only had one period'
- 'I try to lose weight for my boyfriend'
- 'my sister's friend was anorexic, she didn't get periods, she stopped eating to stop her periods'

compared with those of fashionable and popular media personalities. It is significant that, in contrast to older women, adolescent girls perceive their bodies part by part, noting particularly the size and shape of their breasts and the size of their thighs, bottom, hips, and abdomen. The thighs are particularly vulnerable to an overperception of size—the girl perceiving her thighs as larger and uglier than they usually are.

Adolescents' perception of their body size

The overperception of body size is found amongst teenage girls in many countries. In a Swedish study of the entire female population of a small town, in the late 1960s, 26 per cent of 14-year-olds perceived themselves as fat; and among the 18-year-olds, over 50 per cent reported that they were fat. In the USA in the 1970s a study of 1000 teenagers attending high school showed that the girls were particularly preoccupied with their body shape and their weight. About half of them classified themselves as obese, although anthropometric measurements showed that only 25 per cent were obese by the criteria used by the authors, which were based on standard US weight, height, and age tables.

In the mid-1980s, in the USA, 2500 teenage women aged 15 to 18 were surveyed. There had been little change in perceptions about body shape and weight and attitudes to being fat. Forty-three per cent of the girls perceived themselves as overweight and 31 per cent feared that they looked fat. Eighty-two per cent wanted to lose weight, 39 per cent worried about overeating and 18 per cent were fearful they would gain weight.

Another US study made in 1991 confirmed this finding. In this study, 60 per cent of the school students (mean age 16) described themselves as being overweight; 75 per cent wanted to lose weight; 80 per cent said that they were above the weight at which they would be happiest.

Three Australian studies conducted in the 1990s of over 1200 adolescent women reported similar findings. The investigations showed that between one-third and one-half of the teenage women whose weight was normal perceived themselves as overweight.

It is apparent from these studies that the attitudes of young women in these three developed countries about their body shape and weight have not changed in the past three decades.

Faced with this preoccupation about their body shape and weight, it appears that between one-third and two-thirds of all teenage women in the USA and similar developed countries, go on diets and one woman in six diets 'seriously'.

Feelings about body weight and shape after menarche

Young women's concerns about their body weight, body shape, and body appearance increase in the year after their first period (Fig. 4). In response to these worries most women commence dieting or trying to reduce their food intake. A few years later these young teenagers appear to adjust and become more accepting of their increased body weight but not their body shape. Their body image concerns continue to increase along with the psychological changes in anxiety, depression, social unease, and feelings of loss of control following menarche. The development of all these worries, feelings, and dieting behaviour from the time of menarche are shown in Fig. 4.

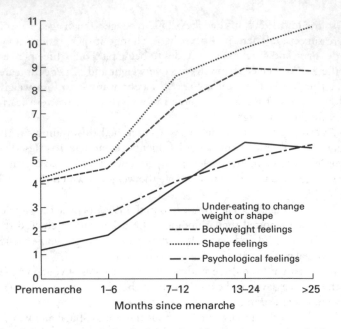

Fig. 4. Increasing negative feelings about body shape and weight and dieting following menarche.

Adolescent and young people's eating behaviour

We have been interested in teenage and young people's eating behaviour for the past 20 years.

In two studies we found evidence to support an association between the menstrual cycle and food intake in young women. There is an increase in the intake of carbohydrates, protein, and fats, and hence of energy in the day or two before and after the onset of menstrual bleeding. Individual women show a wide variation in the amount of food eaten, frequently depending on how women are feeling. Many women have feelings of depression, irritability, and tension just before their period, and enjoy a feeling of well-being and a decrease their appetite in the week after menstruation. It is during these days following bleeding that women find they can successfully reduce their food intake and commence dieting. Later in the menstrual cycle, from ovulation, women find dieting and control around food is more difficult. Usually the greater the food restriction early in the menstrual cycle the more likely craving for food and binge-eating will occur in the premenstrual phase of that menstrual cycle. It is perhaps easier to understand if you think that between ovulation and the next period the body is preparing for a possible pregnancy, it is making a home in the uterus for a baby to grow and develop for the next 40 weeks. The thick engorged lining of the uterus provides nutrients and energy for the embryo when it first arrives in the uterus, before the placenta can transport the nutrients and energy from its mother. A potential mother who is eating adequately is more likely to provide this home for her baby.

The Sydney study showed that the daily quantity of food eaten could vary fourfold. In the Swedish study quoted earlier, one-third of the teenage girls alternated dieting with periods of binge-eating; and such eating behaviour was more common among the older teenage girls.

We also asked four groups of Australian young women aged 15 to 25 to complete a questionnaire about their eating habits, menstrual status, and the behaviour which they used to control their weight. The groups were students, ballet dancers, anorexia nervosa patients, and bulimia nervosa patients. Of the 106 students surveyed, 94 per cent had tried to diet at some time, the majority first trying between the ages of 13 and 18. Seventy-nine per cent said that they wanted to be a little or a lot lighter in weight and 31 per cent said that they had difficulty in controlling their weight.

In 1988 another study of Australian women aged 19 to 29 showed that over 50 per cent had experienced difficulty in controlling their weight at some time. Four out of every ten teenagers considered that they had an ongoing problem of weight control and one in three felt that the problem interfered with their daily lives. Like the Swedish and the American teenagers and young women, most of the Australian women wanted to lose weight from their thighs, bottom, hips, and abdomen (Table 2). Sixty-three per cent of the Australian young women said that they had episodes of overeating when they 'couldn't stop'. Eighteen per cent of the teenagers aged 15 to 18, and 23 per cent of the women aged 18 to 26 were habitual 'binge-eaters'. One woman in ten, aged 18 to 26 considered that binge-eating was a great problem for them. To control their weight most of the Australian young women avoided eating between meals, took energetic exercise, kept busy to avoid the temptation to eat, missed out

Table 2. Areas of the body from which women want to lose weight

	1981 study	1987 study
	Per cent of women	
Thighs	64	75
Bottom	45	65
Hips	43	80
Waist/stomach	22	80
Legs	20	
Face	9	
All over	9	
Breasts	6	
Arms	6	

one (or more) meals each day, chose low-calorie foods, or one of the other methods shown in Table 3.

Many of the 1200 young women (mean age 15) surveyed in the three Australian studies (mentioned on page 9) had disturbed eating behaviour. One-third had been on 'crash diets' or had episodes of fasting, and half 'avoided meals'. Twenty-three per cent of the women had used 'potentially dangerous weight control behaviours' and 10 per cent smoked 'to lose weight'.

The weight control measures described are similar to those used by women who have an eating disorder such as bulimia nervosa or anorexia nervosa.

Disturbed eating behaviour affects young as well as older teenagers. In 1994 the eating behaviours of 200 Australian boys and 300 girls aged 10–14 years old were surveyed. The girls were divided into two groups: those who were prepubertal, that is they had not started menstruating, and those who had passed their menarche. The results showed that 16 per cent of the prepubertal girls and 40 per cent of the girls who had passed their menarche perceived themselves as too fat. Nineteen per cent of the boys also perceived themselves as too fat. In an attempt to control their weight most of those surveyed had used sensible methods of weight control, but 20 per cent of the girls and 9 per cent of the boys used extreme methods, including smoking.

Table 3. Weight-losing behaviour of 300 female teenagers aged 10–14 and 106 healthy women aged 15–25 (per cent using)

	Age	
	10–14	**15–25**
Avoiding eating between meals	73	78
Exercising (usually alone)	44	75
Dieting – 'own diet'	35	55
Avoiding eating breakfast	–	48
Keeping busy to avoid temptation to eat	38	46
Selecting low-kilojoule (calorie) foods	32	41
Counting calories	–	34
Avoiding situations where food is offered	15	25
Dieting with a friend	–	22
Using illness as an excuse not to eat	–	21
Exercising with a friend	–	20
Drinking water before eating	29	18
Taking 'natural' laxatives	11	16
Lying about the amount of food eaten	–	16
Weighing self several times a day	4	15
Smoking cigarettes	2	14
Dieting – magazine diet	16	12
Keeping no food at home	–	12
Avoiding eating with family	1	10

Summary of studies of adolescent eating behaviour

It is evident from these studies that in several Western countries, most young women (and some young men) are unnecessarily concerned about their body shape and believe they have a problem with their weight. These concerns lead them to take measures to lose weight, even though their actual weight is in the normal range. It also appears that anxieties about body shape and weight are being expressed at an earlier age than a decade ago.

How adolescents control their body shape and weight

Although concern about body shape and weight is occurring among younger teenagers, on average, teenage woman first become aware of their body shape and weight in the year after their first menstrual period. About a year later, many young women start trying simple and safe methods of weight control, such as not snacking between meals and exercising. By the age of 15 years young women may start on a diet which they believe will be successful in enabling them to lose weight.

Most women diet for shorter or longer periods, with about a quarter of those who diet doing so 'seriously'. Some women (14–30 per cent) fast for periods of time, usually a day or two, to try to reduce their weight quickly. Some women (25–65 per cent) exercise to lose weight and to change their body shape. About three women in every hundred self-induce vomiting, and between 1 and 5 per cent abuse laxatives (Table 4).

By the age of 17 the minority of adolescent women who are having serious problems with eating, body shape, and body weight, recognize the fact. These women try the various methods of weight control just mentioned but the frequent use of dangerous methods of weight control, such as self-induced vomiting and laxative abuse, does not start until

Table 4. Methods young women in Australia, Britain, and the USA use to lose weight

	per cent
Dieting	20–35
Severe dieting (intermittent starvation)	10–15
Smoking cigarettes	8–15
Diuretics (more than once per week)	0.5–3
Laxative abuse (more than once per week)	1–5
Vomiting	2–8

the young woman is aged 18 on average, and if chosen most young women will have used one or more of them by the age of 22.

As well as restricting food intake and exercising to lose weight, a number of women (variously reported as 14 to 46 per cent) go on eating binges, usually starting at about the age of 18.

Media pressures and dieting

Women of all ages in Western society, but especially those under the age of 40, are subjected to enormous pressures to be slim and look good. A 'perfect' body is equated with high self-esteem, success (in romance and a career), acceptance, and admiration by others. Television advertising sitcoms, and 'soap operas' portray the heroines as slim, young, and beautiful. The cinema, women's magazines, and popular newspapers further encourage the belief that to 'succeed' and be happy women should be slim. In these circumstances it is not surprising that a preoccupation with body shape and size is widespread amongst young women.

Women tend to put on weight as they grow older and women in their 40s and 50s are also responding to these pressures. Many women in these age groups want to have the body shape and weight of a woman in her 20s, encouraged by fashion designers and by advertising in women's magazines. To control their weight gain, many middle-aged women diet or take more exercise, but a few adopt the more dangerous methods of weight control with adverse consequences to their health.

The weight loss industry is thriving. Each year a large number of paperback books are published which extol an 'exciting' new diet. Often these diets are nutritionally unsound, some are dangerous to health. Women's magazines publish articles about diet in almost every issue. The efficacy of the diet books and articles in helping the reader achieve and maintain a reduced weight is questionable as new diets appear so frequently, and disappear just as frequently, to be superseded by another 'fad' diet. It seems that the twenty-first century woman desires a miracle diet which is effective, painless psychologically and physically, and can be adopted with no disturbance to her lifestyle. No such diet exists or can exist. Because of this, many women diet for a while then stop and, after an interval, start a new 'guaranteed' diet. This cycle of yo-yo dieting many continue over a number of years. Recent evidence from the United States suggests that the more diets a person tries the harder it becomes to lose weight. There is also a suggestion that these people are at a greater risk of having a heart attack in middle age.

This pattern of dieting may have other disturbing psychological consequences to the dieter. With weight loss the woman achieves what she desired, at least partially. If the weight is regained during the next few weeks or months, she may become depressed and lose her self-esteem. She begins another attempt to lose weight with another diet and the circle continues.

The barrage of information extolling slim bodies among women induces many women to diet, fast intermittently, or exercise. In spite of (or because of) taking these actions, most young women's weight fluctuates within the 'desirable' range for their height.

As we have reported, studies from Britain, the USA, and Australia show that up to one-third of adolescent women try periods of fasting to control their weight, and one-third of young women binge-eat from time to time. One woman in ten induces vomiting periodically as a means of controlling her weight.

A smaller proportion of young women choose a method or more than one method of weight control which may increase the health risks to the woman. These are some 'fad' diets, starvation, self-induced vomiting, laxative abuse, diuretic and slimming tablet abuse, and smoking.

The safety of 'fad' diets, meal substitutes, and commercial weight-loss programmes depends to a large extent on the person who chooses one or more of the methods. For example, a 'fad' diet which is nutritionally inadequate or dangerous, is harmless if the woman abandons it after a few days; and a commercial weight-loss regimen which is nutritionally sound becomes potentially dangerous if the user seeks to increase her weight loss by alternating the diet with periods of starvation.

Laxative abuse and self-induced vomiting are potentially dangerous methods of weight control. Laxative abuse, that is taking more than twice the recommended dose at least once a week for more than three months, may cause dehydration and in a few cases electrolyte disturbances. As more women have become aware that taking laxatives is an ineffective method of weight control, its use is declining. A recent survey showed that only 2 per cent of women aged 18 or less were using laxatives to control their weight compared with 5 per cent a decade ago.

In contrast, self-induced vomiting seems to be increasing and is commencing at a younger age, as early as 11 years in some cases. Most teenagers who use self-induced vomiting to control their weight do so infrequently, but one teenage woman in 20 induces vomiting more than once a week. Self-induced vomiting may cause dehydration or may damage the girl's teeth as the acid vomit eats into the tooth enamel. It occasionally leads to vomiting blood (haematemesis).

Smoking and body weight

At a time when the health risks of smoking are becoming increasingly apparent, the use of cigarette smoking by young women as a method of weight control is increasing. Recent findings in the UK and USA suggest that the greater the concern a young woman has about her weight the greater is her use of cigarettes. Some young women start cigarette smoking and some older women continue smoking to control their body weight. Studies have shown that up to 37 per cent of young women who smoke, do so to control their body weight. In a study of pregnant women we conducted in 1989, we found that 4 per cent of the pregnant women continued to smoke during pregnancy in order to control their weight gain, in spite of having been advised not to smoke. In a similar group of pregnant women in 1998 fewer women smoked before they were pregnant but 4 per cent continued to smoke to control their weight during pregnancy. Women with an eating disorder, particularly bulimia nervosa, may find it difficult to stop smoking as they fear that if they do their weight will increase.

They have reason to be worried as most women gain weight after ceasing to smoke. A study made in the USA of a large national sample compared the weight gain of continuing smokers with that of people who had quit smoking over a ten-year period. The Body Mass Index or BMI (see page 24) of women smokers increased from 25.5 to 26.5, whilst that of women who had quit smoking increased from 25.5 to 28.0. The average weight gain over the ten-year period among the women who had ceased to smoke was 3.8 kg and among the men 2.8 kg.

Those people who were under the age of 55 and who smoked 15 or more cigarettes a day were more likely to gain weight. The authors of the study concluded: 'Weight gain is not likely to negate the health benefits of smoking cessation, but its cosmetic effects may interfere with attempts to quit.'

We believe that this is especially so among women who have an eating disorder.

It is now thought that the weight gain after quitting smoking is returning a person to their normal body weight. Why tobacco smoking results in an artificially lowered body weight is thought to arise from a variety of physiological and psychological reasons. Smoking may be a psychological substitute for eating. Nicotine is thought to help improve depressed moods and suppress appetite by its action on chemical transmitter substances, such as serotonin, in the brain. Although not confirmed in people, when laboratory rats are given nicotine they decrease both the number of meals they eat and the amount eaten at each meal. Nicotine also increases the basal metabolic rate (BMR) of men and women, probably by increasing the amount of fat, protein, and glycogen used by the body and decreasing the amount of glucose taken into tissues of the body. This occurs because nicotine reduces the amount of the hormone, insulin, released after food is eaten. An increase in BMR without an increase in additional energy in the form of food intake will result in weight decrease. The stimulatory effect of nicotine may also contribute to the overall lower body weight of smokers.

The results of studies of exercise programs, nicotine patches, and the newer antidepressant medications (serotonin reuptake inhibitors) aimed to prevent weight gain and improve cessation of smoking rates are unclear at this time.

Binge-eating and the eating disorders

Some young women intersperse periods of strict dieting by episodes of uncontrollable overeating, or binge-eating, probably because their body responds to the lack of food by altering its physiology. The changes in diet send messages to a centre in the brain which increases the physiological pressure to eat, and often to overeat or binge. In most cases the eating binges are infrequent and do not affect the young woman's quality of life or her lifestyle. In some cases her quality of life is affected and she loses control over her eating behaviour, which may result in the development of the binge-eating disorder or of bulimia nervosa, which may disrupt the life of the woman consider ably and, if dangerous methods of weight control—self-induced vomiting and laxative or diuretic abuse—are used, may lead to serious illness.

Other young women are so concerned about losing control of their eating behaviour that they starve themselves and start on a relentless pursuit of thinness. They eat minimal amounts of food, and many use the dangerous methods of weight control mentioned earlier. The result is that they become emaciated and their menstrual periods cease. They develop anorexia nervosa.

Although these two disorders predominantly affect young women in Western countries, recent research shows that the same problems are becoming increasingly diagnosed among all social classes and ethnic groups. For example, the eating disorders are being diagnosed amongst young women in Japan and some other Asian countries.

Those teenagers who choose to ignore the social pressures to become and to remain thin, and continue eating more energy than they need for their bodily functions, gain weight progressively and become obese. In fact a person who is grossly obese (see Fig. 8 on p. 29) has at least 1260 MJ (300 000 kcals) of energy stored in her body as fat.

The outcome of the young woman's concern about her body shape and her disordered eating behaviour is shown in Fig. 5. The disordered eating behaviour usually starts between the ages of 14 and 18.

We would stress that the binge-eating disorder, anorexia nervosa, bulimia nervosa, and obesity (especially morbid obesity)—are not *illnesses* in themselves. They become illnesses when they interfere with the person's physical or mental comfort; of if they are likely to produce more medical complications; or disorganize the person's life to a marked degree; or so distort her or his life that close relatives are also involved and help is sought. Unfortunately, in severe cases, unless treatment is sought the eating disorder may lead to the premature death of the victim.

Pregnancy and eating behaviour

Although most eating disorder problems start in adolescence, a further challenge to some women's attitude to weight, body image, exercise, and eating behaviour may occur when they become pregnant.

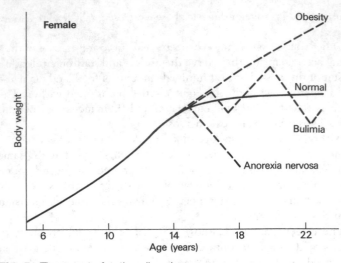

Fig. 5. The onset of eating disorders.

We have studied the attitudes of 100 healthy pregnant women admitted consecutively to a teaching hospital to give birth to their first child. We questioned the women three to five days after the birth about their eating and weight control behaviours at any stage in their life before they became pregnant and during the pregnancy.

Before the pregnancy, the proportion of the women using methods of weight-losing behaviour, and the methods used, were similar to those used by the 106 normal, healthy non-pregnant women whose behaviours we have reported on page 13.

During the pregnancy, 71 of the women 'watched their weight', 52 reported that thoughts of food interfered with their concentration (eight reporting that this was a severe problem) and 41 women said that they had had problems controlling their weight gain. Forty-four of the women reported binge-eating (the same proportion as before pregnancy) and nine (three times as many as before pregnancy) said that they considered their binge-eating to be severe.

Because of their concern about weight gain, which may have been increased by the advice that they were receiving from their doctor, many of the women used one or more ways of controlling their weight gain. Most of the methods adopted were sensible. For example, nearly half of the pregnant women reduced their food intake modestly by choosing low energy foods, by avoiding eating between meals, by 'counting calories', or by exercising sensibly. Most of these women had used similar methods to control their weight before becoming pregnant. Eleven women adopted one or more methods of weight control which had the potential to harm their baby or themselves. Four of the 11 women took excessive exercise, four continued smoking cigarettes, three periodically starved themselves, two abused laxatives, and one woman self-induced vomiting throughout the pregnancy.

This study shows that many women who do not have an eating disorder are concerned about weight gain, body image, and eating behaviour in pregnancy.

Most women meet this challenges and adjust to the changes of pregnancy, childbirth, breast-feeding, and parenthood. Most women who have 'normal eating patterns' feel they improve their eating patterns and nutrition during pregnancy as they wish to care for their developing child. Being concerned about gaining body weight and the possibility of not losing this weight after the birth is a common concern of pregnancy. The experiences of pregnant women suffering from eating disorders are discussed in Chapter 5.

2 Eating disorders—an overview

The human being is an open social system, each one, in its own way unique. My food problem is my somewhat unique reaction to a board of external and internal influences. Human beings prefer things in a state of organization, they dislike randomness and attempt to classify.

The control of eating

The control of normal eating behaviour is not well understood. Although more is known about the many factors that influence the control of food intake it is still puzzling how they all fit together. The discovery of leptin is an important recent advancement as this hormone is involved in the energy balance in the body of humans. Leptin is a hormone that tells the body when you are satiated and do not need further food. It is secreted by fat (adipose) tissue and reflects the amount of energy stored in the body as fat. Receptors in the hypothalamus of the brain are sensitive to the levels of leptin and regulate the amount of body fat by controlling the appetite and increasing energy output. The most potent appetite stimulant in the brain is called neuropeptide Y (NPY); leptin suppresses the stimulation of appetite by NPY. Other hormones from the stomach, intestines, and bloodstream in turn regulate leptin. How the sight, smell, and taste sensations associated with food are integrated with the chemical and neural messages received by the brain is unclear as these sensations may encourage or discourage eating. Eating can be influenced in other ways in human beings.

Cultural beliefs about foods also affect eating behaviour in various ways. For example, the Chinese eat dog meat, Europeans eat horse meat, Americans add sugar or syrup to many foods, the British and Australians eat meat pies—all foods which some other cultures either reject or dislike. To some extent this cultural diversity of food preferences is changing as increasing numbers of people in many countries are enjoying fast foods from multinational outlets. A further factor affecting eating behaviour is mood. People who are depressed usually eat far less, whilst people who are anxious may relieve their anxiety by eating food. Women with eating disorders often believe 'you are what you eat' and believe that they can control their body weight and shape by the food they eat. In fact, nearly all the energy derived from foodstuffs is converted into heat that is used to keep the cells of the body warm so each cell can carry out the work it is designed to do to help the body function as a whole. What receptors in the brain keep body weight so surprisingly stable in most individuals is unknown. We do know that increased levels of leptin in the blood decrease food intake and increase the body's activity and heat production. What is also known is that these mechanisms and receptors fail to function when they are over or under stimulated by starvation or gorging. Women with eating disorders find their perceptions of hunger and satiation (fullness) are not to be believed. Somehow these messages from the brain are scrambled by their behaviours. Studies have shown disturbances in the release of hormones affecting appetite in these patients.

The levels of leptin in the bloodstream also reflect the amount of energy stored as fat in the adipose tissue of the body and not just in the hours following a meal. The levels are higher in men and women with greater body fat. It has been hypothesized that obesity that is not due to excess energy intake may result from a genetic change that prevents the production of leptin. It is also thought that leptin may play a part in the so-called body weight 'set point' concept. Recent research shows that people have a different 'set point' for their body weight. It is thought this is determined by a network of neurons in several parts of the brain which are collectively called the adipostat.

Defining an ideal weight

A number of calculations have been used to define maximum and minimum ideal weights. The simplest is a measurement of weight against height, as used by insurance companies (Fig. 7). If a woman has lost at least 25 per cent of her weight by this scale, she is defined as anorexic. A more sophisticated measure takes into account the person's age, as well as weight and height, as obtained from a table prepared by the Society of Actuaries and is called the Average Body Weight (ABW).

The Body Mass Index is the third type of calculation, and the one used in this book. Devised in 1871 by a Belgian astronomer and mathematician, Dr Quetelet, for defining obesity, it is equally valuable in reaching a diagnosis of anorexia nervosa. The *Quetelet Index*, which is now known as the *Body Mass Index* (BMI) is calculated from the simple formula W/H^2, that is:

$$\frac{\text{weight in kilograms}}{\text{height in metres} \times \text{height in metres}}$$

The person is weighed in indoor clothing without shoes (Fig. 8, p. 29). A table of heights and corresponding BMI values is in the Appendix to this book (pages 300–66).

The various eating disorders, as in most other psychosomatic conditions, have slightly different classifications. However we can give a general definition for each disorder by putting together features most commonly described.

Anorexia nervosa

People may find it hard to believe or comprehend why a person, supposedly intelligent and quite attractive and with a good family upbringing would throw it all away for an obsessive need—no, desire!—to be slender and praised for the will-power to diet so well and easily.

The term anorexia nervosa was first used by an English physician, Sir William Gull, in 1873. He described a young woman, 'Miss A', whom he had first seen seven years earlier:

Her emaciation was very great. It was stated that she had lost 33 lbs. in weight. She was then 5 st. 12 lbs. Height, 5 ft. 5 in. Amenorrhoea for nearly a year. No cough. Respirations throughout chest everywhere normal. Heart sounds normal. Resp. 12; pulse, 56. No vomiting nor diarrhoea. Slight constipation. Complete anorèxia for animal food, and almost complete anorexia for everything else. Abdomen shrunk and flat, collapsed. No abnormal pulsations of aorta. Tongue clean. Urine normal. Slight deposit of phosphates on boiling. The condition was one of simple starvation. There was but slight variation in her condition, though observed at intervals of three or four months . . . The case was regarded as one of simple anorexia.

Various remedies were prescribed—the preparations of cinchona, the bichloride of mercury, syrup of the iodide of orion, syrup of the phosphate of iron, citrate of quinine and iron, etc., but no perceptible effect followed their administration. The diet also was varied, but without any effect upon the appetite. Occasionally for a day or two the appetite was voracious, but this was very rare and exceptional. The patient complained of no pain, but was restless and active. This was in fact a striking expression of the nervous state, for it seemed hardly possible that a body so wasted could undergo the exercise which seemed agreeable. There was some peevishness of temper, and a feeling of jealousy. No account could be given of the exciting cause. Miss A remained under my observation from January 1866 to March 1868, when she had much improved, and gained weight from 82 to 128 lbs. The improvement from this time continued, and I saw no more of her medically . . . The want of appetite is, I believe, due to a morbid mental state. I have not observed in these cases any gastric disorder to which the want of appetite could be referred. I believe, therefore, that its origin is central and not peripheral. That mental states may destroy appetite is notorious, and it will be admitted that young women at the ages named are specially abnoxious to mental perversity. We might call the state hysterical without committing ourselves to the etymological value of the word, or maintaining that the subjects of it have the common symptoms of hysteria. I prefer, however, the more general term 'nervosa', since the disease occurs in males as well as females, and is probably rather central than peripheral. The importance of discriminating such cases in practice is obvious; otherwise prognosis will be erroneous, and treatment misdirected.

Sir William was in error: anorexia nervosa patients do not have a lack of appetite. They are often hungry, but suppress their hunger and refuse to eat normally, because of their relentless desire to be thin, even to the point of becoming emaciated, and because of their fear that they will lose control of their eating behaviour. Diagnostic criteria are given in Table 5.

The main features of anorexia nervosa

- An *intense fear of becoming fat*. The woman is abnormally sensitive about being fat, or has a morbid fear of becoming fat, and

Table 5. Diagnostic criteria for anorexia nervosa

- has a intense ear of gaining weight or becoming fat, even though she is underweight;
- refuses to maintain her body weight in the normal weight range for her age and height, which is not due to any physical or mental disorder;
- has a body mass index equal to or less than 17.5;
- has a disturbance in her perception of her body weight, size, or shape;
- denies the serious nature of her current low body weight;
- if she has entered her reproductive years (i.e. has passed puberty), has had no menstrual periods (amenorrhoea) for at least three consecutive months.

Two types of anorexia nervosa are indentified. In the first or *restricting type*, the woman restricts her food intake to a very low level and does not regularly engage in binge-eating or purging behaviour. In the second type, the *binge-eating/purging type*, although the woman usually restricts her food intake, she regularly engages in binge-eating and/or purging behaviour, by inducing vomiting or misusing laxatives or diuretics.

Modified from the American Psychiatric Association: Diagnostic and Statistical and Manual of Mental Disorders, 4th edition (1994), American Psychiatric Association, Washington DC. By permission.

of losing her control over the amount of food she eats. This fear induces her to adopt behaviour aimed at losing weight. Most anorexia nervosa victims drastically reduce the amount of food they eat, particularly reducing food rich in fat and carbohydrate. They frequently tend towards vegetarianism, with the elimination of red meat often being reported. This coincides with the onset of restrictive eating and usually weight loss. Some anorexics use other methods of weight reduction, in addition to limiting the food they eat. The behaviours vary, but self-induced vomiting, the use of excessive amounts of laxatives or diuretics, and strenuous exercise are the most common.

- *Weight loss.* When presenting to a doctor the woman has usually lost a considerable amount of weight, so that her BMI is 17.5 or below. An obvious source of diagnostic error could creep in here. For example, women who have severe psychotic mental illness may believe that their food is poisoned, refuse to eat, and suffer considerable weight loss. Or the woman may be depressed and react by avoid-

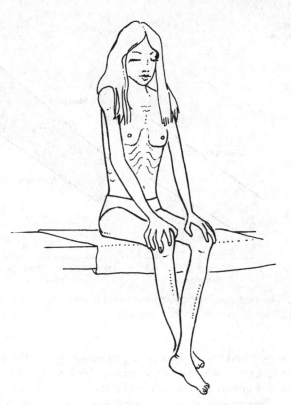

Fig. 6. A young woman suffering from anorexia nervosa.

ing eating, because she cannot be bothered to eat. Marked physical diseases, such as terminal cancer and tuberculosis, may be associated with extreme emaciation. For these reasons, the woman must have no other physical or psychological illness, which might account for her loss in weight, before a diagnosis of anorexia nervosa is made. Once a physical or a mental illness has been excluded, a woman whose BMI is less than 17.5 may have anorexia nervosa.

As mentioned above, various weight/height measures may be used in the diagnosis of anorexia nervosa. If she is below 45 kg, has lost at least 25 per cent of her 'ideal' or desirable body weight as calculated as shown in Figure 7, or if her weight is less than 85 per cent of the ABW, she may have anorexia nervosa.

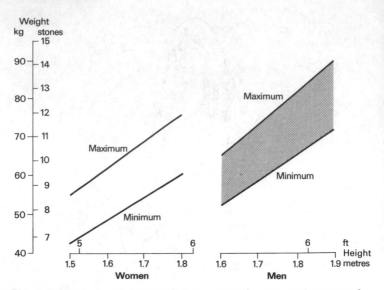

Fig. 7. Maximum and minimum ideal weights for men and women of different heights, wearing indoor clothing.

We have found BMI to be a more precise measure of the degree of underweight or emaciation. If the person's BMI is between 17.5 and 18.5 she is definitely underweight and if the other criteria mentioned in this section are present she may have an eating disorder. If her BMI is 17.5 or below and she is not a famine victim and has no mental or physical illness, she probably has anorexia nervosa. However, the BMI of prepubertal women must be interpreted carefully as no accurate BMI tables, which include age, are available. Teenage girls who have not started menstruating have lower BMIs than girls of the same age who have reached their menarche. The BMI of female school students before and after their first menstrual period is shown in Chapter one p. 5.

 • *Lack of menstruation.* The third feature common to most descriptions of anorexia nervosa is that a girl who has started to menstruate ceases menstruating—she develops amenorrhoea. Amenorrhoea may occur early in the illness before any great loss of weight has occurred, and menstruation invariably is absent in emaciated women. In fact most women cease to menstruate when their weight is in the BMI range of 17–19. If a woman is taking the oral contraceptive 'pill' or 'hormone replacement' this feature cannot be determined. Women taking 'the pill' will bleed because the hormones are withdrawn, this is not menstruation, this is called 'withdrawal bleeding'. A woman taking 'the pill' who is at low weight will not know if she has amenorrhoea until she ceases taking 'the pill'. A few women, particularly older women with established menstrual cycles, will menstruate at a BMI below 17.

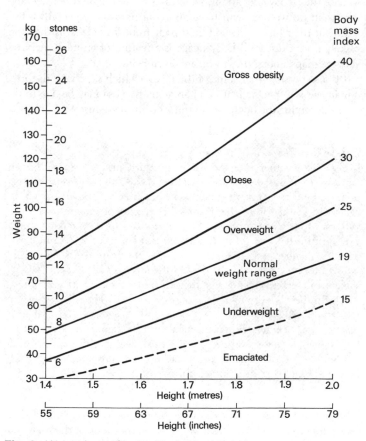

Fig. 8. Weight/height^2 index (Body Mass Index).

Distorted body image

Some experts claim that a distorted body image—the woman perceiving her body as larger, wider, and fatter than it is in reality—is a specific feature of anorexia nervosa. This is inaccurate as many other women, such as pregnant women, who have recently changed their body shape, have the same disturbed body-image. It is true that many severely emaciated women suffering from anorexia nervosa lose insight into how emaciated they are; in other words, they deny their thinness. These women have a grossly distorted perception of their body size. But it is also known that many women who have normal eating behaviour over-estimate their body size, and in some cases overestimate it considerably more than do women who have anorexia nervosa, especially when looking at their hip width and their body from the side. It is therefore unlikely that a distorted body image is a feature of anorexia nervosa, except perhaps among those who are severely ill.

It is also possible that some of the reports which say that a distorted body image is a specific feature of anorexia nervosa may be due to the patient deceiving the doctor, as in the following case history.

Case history: Clara
I've spoken to other anorexics and they realize just as I realize that at our lowest weights, we all knew we were damn thin. You'd have to be pretty stupid to think that you were not, but you have to hide it because if you let on to the doctors that you know you are thin, they will want to put weight on you. So you keep letting on you don't think you are thin but you think you are normal and they will think your way. I remember two anorexics who were so sincere to the Professor, telling him they were normal. I asked them if they felt like me, falsely sincere and secretive. They said they did. How could they think otherwise with their bones sticking out of their bottoms. The next day when I saw the Professor he said 'Clara, do you think you are thin?' My first reaction was 'see, he doesn't know, he must be dumb. Oh, I won't tell him though, because I want to stay like this: I feel safe, out of the world and men are too scared to touch me in case they break me.' So I answered him 'Of course I'm not thin.'

Women who have anorexia nervosa tend to look at parts of their body, rather than their body as a whole, when they look at themselves in a mirror. They see their abdomen as 'bulgy' and they want it to be flat.

They perceive their thighs as ungainly, large, and heavy, and want them to be smooth and thinner. These perceptions also occur to normal women, as we found when we asked several groups of women the question: 'What would you prefer your weight to be?' The groups were of women who were students, ballet dancers, or women with eating disorders. Each of the groups wanted to be thinner (Table 6).

When the perceptions of body image by a woman who has anorexia nervosa are further analysed, it becomes apparent that what the woman was saying was that when her weight was normal she saw parts of her body, for example her thighs, as too heavy, and, although she was now emaciated, she still saw her thighs as heavier and bigger than the rest of her body. In other words, although she knew that she was thin she *felt* that she was fat.

These features have been discussed by a Committee of the American Psychiatric Association who have developed criteria for the diagnosis of anorexia nervosa (Table 5). The criteria indicate that there are two types of anorexia nervosa.

1. *Anorexia nervosa—restricting type* or *dieters*. This affects 60 per cent of sufferers, who lose weight primarily by dieting, fasting, or taking excessive exercise, or all of these methods. Occasionally they misuse laxatives.

2. *Anorexia nervosa—binge-eating/purging type* or *vomiters and purgers*. These women have episodes of binge-eating and try to prevent the food being absorbed by self-induced vomiting and/or the abuse of purgatives or enemas. In these behaviours they resemble women who have bulimia nervosa.

Table 6. What young women would like their weight to be

	Healthy women (106)	Ballet dancers (50)	Anorexia nervosa patients (22)	Bulimia nervosa patients (44)
			Per cent	
A lot heavier	0	1	9	0
A little heavier	1	1	50	0
Present weight	17	3	5	14
A little lighter	47	60	23	18
A lot lighter	32	30	14	64

Bulimia nervosa

Looking back on the reason I started binge-eating, I think it was because of my obsession with dieting. And that stemmed from the fact that I thought I was overweight when in reality I was short and had inherited fatter arms and legs than the average person.

Bulimia means to eat like an ox. Although people have been known to 'eat like oxen' from antiquity, it was not until 1979 that a London psychiatrist, Gerald Russell, identified a number of his anorexia nervosa patients who had an 'ominous variation' of the disorder, the variation being that they periodically went on eating binges.

Subsequent studies showed that although about 40 per cent of anorexia nervosa patients episodically binge-ate, people who did not have anorexia nervosa binge-ate frequently (more than twice a week) and persisted in the behaviour for more than three months.

It became clear that these patients had a separate eating disorder which was given the name bulimia, and later called bulimia nervosa. This is not the same as the binge-eating disorder; the sufferers, as well as feeling that they have a lack of control over their eating behaviour, binge-eat very frequently, and adopt measures, some of which are dangerous to their health, to prevent them becoming increasingly fat.

Most of the patients were women. They divided their days into 'good days' when they had no compulsion to binge-eat, and 'bad days' when they found the need to binge-eat irresistible. They were also aware that anxiety, boredom, stress, or unhappiness could precipitate an episode of binge-eating.

The increasing interest in bulimia nervosa, which is four to six times as common as anorexia nervosa, persuaded the American College of Psychiatrists to develop criteria for the diagnosis of the eating disorder (Table 7).

Bulimia nervosa patients know that they have an eating disorder. They are fascinated by food and buy cook-books and read magazine articles about food and cooking. They enjoy discussing food and diets, and often use eating as a way of escaping from the unpleasant stresses of life, to the extent that they have an all-consuming desire to eat. But they are aware that binge-eating is quite distinct from overeating. Between binges they may diet rigorously, and may try to resist the urge to binge-eat, rather as an alcoholic tries to resist the urge to drink. This analogy may be more exact than is obvious at first sight, as at least 20 per cent of bulimia patients abuse alcohol or drugs.

Table 7. Diagnostic criteria for bulimia nervosa

The woman:
- has recurrent episodes of binge-eating, that is she rapidly consumes a large amount of food (binge-eating) in a short period of time (usually less than two hours);
- feels that she lacks control over her eating behaviour during the eating binges;
- regularly engages in measures to prevent gaining weight, such as self-induced vomiting, laxative misuse or diuretics, strict dieting, fasting, or vigorous exercise;
- has had a minimum average of two binge-eating episodes a week (and the weight-gain prevention measures) for at least three months;
- has a persistent over-concern with her body shape and weight;
- the eating disturbance does not occur exclusively in association with anorexia nervosa.

Eating disorder experts divide bulimia nervosa sufferers into two groups. The first group, '*the purging subtype*', are those women who mainly compensate for their binge-eating eating behaviour by vomiting and purging. The second group, '*the non-purging subtype*', are those women who restrict their food intake (including fasting) between binge-eating episodes or take excessive exercise, but do not regularly induce vomiting or misuse laxatives.

Modified from the American Psychiatric Association: Diagnostic and Statistical Manual of Mental Disorders, 4th edition (1994), American Psychiatric Association, Washington DC. By permission

During an eating-binge (which usually lasts a few minutes or hours but may go on for days) the woman's resistance to eating fails, and she has an irresistible desire to eat. This leads her to ingest excessive amounts of food, far more than she needs to maintain good nutrition and far more than most other people in her culture normally eat. This causes her to be secretive about her binge-eating, at least in the early stages of the illness. She perceives binge-eating as a very private affair, and plans the binges secretively. It may sound bizarre, but in many cases the woman's husband, or partner, or her parents are unaware that she has been binge-eating three or more times a week for a number of years. Many of the women have a safe place where they can binge privately, and where, if they induce vomiting, they can vomit without discovery. When it becomes known by her parents, her partner, or close friends that she binge-eats, attempts to prevent her binge-eating may be met by hostility; or those close to her may condone her behaviour, in the hope that she will stop. As a woman who has bulimia nervosa is aware that binge-eating and overeating are distinct, and because she has a fear of putting on weight, she takes measures to make sure that the food she has eaten during an eating-binge will not lead to a weight increase. To achieve this she may adopt one or more of several methods. She may diet strictly or starve between eating-binges or she may exercise excessively, spending hours each day in the gymnasium, or jogging, playing squash, or swimming. If she finds that these measures do not control her weight, she may resort to a more dangerous method of weight reduction by making sure that the food she eats is not absorbed. She may achieve this by inducing herself to vomit or by taking large amounts of laxatives in the belief that the food she has eaten will not be absorbed.

More than half of bulimia nervosa patients induce vomiting during and at the end of each eating-binge, and all binge-eaters try to diet between binges, although many fail to keep to their chosen diet. A minority of binge-eaters do not induce vomiting and maintain a very strict diet between eating-binges, controlling their weight in this way. They find that eating 'anything' leads to binge-eating and they alternate starvation with binge-eating. Some bulimia nervosa patients also abuse laxatives or diuretics between binges in an attempt to keep their weight under control.

There are considerable variations in the weight-losing behaviour of binge-eaters, but, in general, 'vomiters' tend to have a longer history of binge-eating and to take more time in preparing food for the binge. They also seem to have a greater degree of 'feeling good' after a binge than non-vomiters, who are more likely to feel guilty or sad. In other words the feelings of unhappiness, anxiety, or stress which precipitated an eating-binge are relieved to a greater extent among those bulimia nervosa patients who induce vomiting than among those who use other behaviours to avoid weight gain. Some bulimic patients find that vomiting gives them so much 'relief' that they binge-eat in order to vomit.

Anorexia nervosa not for weight and shape (ANNWS)

Anorexia nervosa not for weight or shape (ANNWS) is not an official diagnosis. It is introduced in this book to allow women, frequently young women, to receive help for an eating disorder that does not fit into other classifications. Anorexia nervosa, bulimia nervosa, and EDNOS (discussed later in this chapter) assume the woman has a desire for change or control of body weight and shape. A large part of treatment of these 'dieting disorders' involves concerns about body image.

Anorexia nervosa not for weight and shape includes those women who are not excessively concerned about their body appearance or body weight, who lose weight and maintain low body weight. They resemble women with anorexia nervosa in all aspects of the illness except those relating to body shape and weight. The average examination scores from the Eating and Exercise Examination (EEE) reveal the similarities and differences between sufferers of anorexia nervosa, anorexia nervosa not for weight and shape, and women without an eating disorder (Table 8).

Sufferers worry about eating and control of their eating. They feel preoccupied with food, read and check food labels before buying food and know the nutritional content of most foods. They spend time thinking about what and how much they will eat and what they have

Table 8. Differences and similarities between sufferers of anorexia nervosa, anorexia nervosa not for weight and shape and women without an eating disorder

	Anorexia nervosa N = 32	Anorexia nervosa *not* for weight or shape N = 22	No and eating disorder N = 112
Age (years)	20	19	22
BMI	15	15	22
Undereating for weight or shape	15	8	4
Undereating for any reason	15	12	5
Feelings about weight	15	7	6
Feelings about shape	17	11	8
Attitudes to exercise	14	12	7
Psychological feelings	14	12	4

EEE Examination scores (minimum score 0, maximum score 20)

eaten. They will not eat prepared foods unless they have been involved in the preparation, or if the content is clearly labeled. They feel 'good' when they eat foods they allow themselves and 'bad' if they eat other foods, particularly 'high fat' or 'unhealthy' foods. Women suffering from anorexia nervosa not for weight and shape explain that their aim is to be 'healthy' and/or to be 'fit', to feel better or to control their moods. They change their eating behaviour to allow themselves to eat only healthy food and no fat. Some will explain about learning fat is bad for you in school nutrition classes, they understand (mistakenly) that no fat in the diet is better than some fat or may feel a sense of achievement if they can achieve a diet with no fat. Women may also become preoccupied with exercise and fitness in their pursuit of health. They do not induce vomiting probably as they are not interested in weight loss and wish to maintain a healthy body. Why these women show so little concern about their weight loss is not understood. They recognize some loss of weight but feel being at a lower weight is healthy.

Women who have had anorexia nervosa for many years, who maintain low body weight and have perfect control over their weight sometimes describe losing interest in shape and weight and maintain their eating disorder for other reasons. Young women with anorexia nervosa not for weight or shape may find themselves trapped into maintaining low weight and develop anorexia nervosa. The reason for recognizing anorexia nervosa not for weight and shape but as a separate diagnosis from anorexia nervosa is mainly to allow young people to find help early in their illness before they fulfill the diagnostic criteria for anorexia nervosa. Other benefits are to help therapists plan treatment

Table 9. Possible criteria for anorexia nervosa not for weight or shape, ANNWS.

The woman:
- Has an intense fear of eating food even though she is depriving her body of energy and nutrients;

- Refuses to eat a diet that will provide for her body's needs;

- Has a body mass index BMI below or equal to 17.5;

- Has a disturbance in her perception of what is normal eating for her body weight and energy expenditure;

- Denies the serious nature of her eating behaviour.

that is appropriate for women who are not preoccupied with body shape and weight issues and to avoid sufferers feeling that because they not excessively concerned about body image their therapists 'do not understand them' or 'are not interested in them'. To avoid introducing another new eating disorder it may be appropriate for anorexia nervosa not for weight and shape to be added to eating disorders not otherwise specified (EDNOS) diagnosis that is described later in this chapter.

Binge-eating disorder (BED)

From time to time many people binge-eat (see bulimia nervosa). Usually these people have engaged in periods of strict dieting before they start binge-eating. It is not known why people binge-eat and several other reasons have been suggested in addition to a history of episodes of strict dieting. These include anxiety, concern over a relationship, family problems, depression, or boredom. Research has not yet revealed a conclusive explanation, although as mentioned above the physiological changes resulting from strict dieting or the psychological changes associated with negative moods may cause the release of chemicals in the brain leading to an eating binge.

Because in most cases binge-eating does not affect one's quality of life, medical help is not often sought; however in a few cases the person's life is affected and he or she develops a binge-eating disorder (BED), and then seeks help. Some people seek help for their obesity and the medical problems associated with obesity and do not recognize they are suffering from a binge-eating disorder.

By definition people with a binge-eating disorder do not have anorexia nervosa as their weight is more than BMI 17.5 (see p. 24). Neither do they have bulimia nervosa because they do not regularly use dangerous methods of weight control such as starvation, self-induced vomiting, and laxative abuse. Between 10 and 30 per cent of obese people indulge in binge-eating sufficiently frequently to be classified as having a binge-eating disorder (Table 10).

Some experts believe the diagnosis of binge-eating disorder should not be made unless a person is overweight (BMI greater than 25) or obese (BMI greater than 30). However, many experts do not accept the diagnosis of a specific binge-eating disorder, believing that the cases should be included in the category 'Eating disorders, not otherwise specified (EDNOS); which we will discuss later in this chapter.

Table 10. Proposed diagnostic criteria for the binge-eating disorder

- The woman has recurrent episodes of binge-eating, i.e. eats a substantial amount of food in a short time, usually within two hours. The amount of food is much larger than most people would eat during this time.

- She lacks control over her eating during the binge-eating episode, i.e. she feels that she can't stop eating or control what and how much she eats.

- The binge-eating episodes are associated with a least three of the following:
  (1) she eats much more rapidly than usual;
  (2) she eats until she feels uncomfortably full;
  (3) she eats large amounts of food when not feeling hungry;
  (4) she eats alone, because she is embarrassed about how much she is eating;
  (5) she feels disgusted with herself, depressed, or very guilty about over-eating.

- She is very distressed with regard to her binge-eating.

- The binge-eating occurs, on average, at least two days a week for six months or more.

- The eating behaviour does not occur exclusively during the course of anorexia nervosa or bulimia nervosa.

Modified from the American Psychiatric Association: Diagnostic and Statistical and Manual of Mental Disorders, 4th edition (1994), American Psychiatric Association, Washington DC. By permission.

Atypical eating disorders (EDNOS)

Physicians who specialize in evaluating and treating patients with possible eating disorders have become aware that some of their patients have many, but not all, of the diagnostic criteria of bulimia nervosa or anorexia nervosa necessary to make a diagnosis of either. For example, some women binge-eat huge amounts of food, but only do so once a week. Other women have most of the features of anorexia nervosa, but their body weight is above the range necessary for diagnosis.

A further problem in diagnosis is that some women can be best described as 'chaotic eaters', with a seemingly unpredictable collection of eating and weight-losing behaviours. These women have no idea of 'normal' eating patterns or of the appropriate amount of food necessary for health and to maintain a steady weight.

These groups of women have been classified by the American Psychiatric Association as having an 'eating disorder not otherwise specified' (EDNOS), which is also called 'an atypical eating disorder' (Table 11).

Women with an atypical eating disorder recognize that they have disordered patterns of eating, that they are preoccupied with thoughts of food and body weight and they are aware that their eating disorder affects and interferes with their daily life.

Some of the young women falling into this category of eating dis-order may be in the process of developing all the features needed for a diagnosis of bulimia nervosa or anorexia nervosa, or may be in the process of recovering from one or other of these disorders when first seen. Other women may have avoided developing all the diagnostic criteria for anorexia nervosa or bulimia nervosa but have become obsessed with exercise. They exercise excessively and are developing an 'exercise disorder'.

Several studies have shown that 30 per cent of healthy young women in the community, when questioned, said that they had had an episode of disordered eating, and more than half of them said that they had had recurring episodes over a period of 12 months. Half of these women, when questioned, said that their disordered eating had

Table 11. Atypical eating disorders not otherwise specified (EDNOS)

- If female: all the criteria for anorexia nervosa are met, except that the woman menstruates regularly.

- All the criteria for anorexia nervosa are met except that, despite significant weight loss, the person's current weight is in the normal range.

- All the criteria for bulimia nervosa are met except that the binge-eating and inappropriate behaviours (i.e. purging, laxative abuse, etc.) occur less than twice a week or for a duration of less than three months.

- The person's weight is in the normal range, but she regularly induces vomiting after eating small amounts of food.

- The person repeatedly chews and spits out large amounts of food rather than swallowing the food.

NOTE

Anorexia nervosa *not for weight and shape* is not currently classified as EDNOS. The binge-eating disorder is currently classified as EDNOS.
Modified from the American Psychiatric Association: Diagnostic and Statistical Manual of Mental Disorders, 4th edition (1994) American Psychiatric Association, Washington DC. By permission.

caused them problems and 23 per cent of those aged 18 or more considered their preoccupation with body shape to be a problem. These women are more likely than the others to adopt dangerous methods of weight control. At any one time 8 to 12 per cent of young women can probably be classified as EDNOS.

Women with atypical eating disorders need help from health professionals and community services. Such help may prevent the development of bulimia nervosa or anorexia nervosa in the future. Their concerns should be taken seriously. The criteria for EDNOS are expected to change in the future. The criteria can be made more detailed or more general to include everyone who feels they are suffering from an eating disorder, other than anorexia nervosa and bulimia nervosa. More specific criteria will help researchers understand the different subtypes of EDNOS and develop specific treatment programmes for these different types. Anorexia nervosa not for weight and shape and binge-eating disorder are possible examples. Treatment is usually more acceptable and successful if sufferers feel it is relevant to them.

Obesity

There is considerable controversy among nutritionists as to whether obesity can be classified as an eating disorder. The problem is that people whose weight is 'normal' often eat erratically, sometimes putting on weight, sometimes losing weight. Recently a study was made of over 5000 food choices at various restaurants, snack bars, and cafes. The conclusion of the study was that the major influence on how much people ate was *where* they ate, and that obese people had as wide a range of eating behaviour as 'normal' people; between 10 and 30 per cent had episodes of binge-eating at least twice a week. On the other hand many researchers have shown that obese people choose to eat more food and eat it more quickly than non-obese people. Other researchers have argued that obesity, and particularly severe (or morbid) obesity, occurs in people with a psychiatric problem. However, a study of severely obese people in the United States showed that anxiety, depression, low self-esteem, and poor body image reported by severely obese people were a result, rather than a cause, of their obesity. The study added support to the theory that severe obesity is a habitual disturbance of eating. The experience of nutritionists who try to induce severely obese people to lose weight also suggests that obesity is an eating disorder.

Recently it has been found that there may be a genetic reason for some people becoming obese. It is thought that they have a genetically determined higher 'set-point' for appetite and food intake, in other words they eat more before feeling full (see also page 248), which makes it difficult for them to achieve 'normal' weight.

Reasons for losing weight

The first decision a severely obese person has to make is that she wants to lose weight, either because she finds her body unattractive, or because others remark about her obesity, or because she learns that obesity is dangerous to her health, or that it is aggravating an existing disease such as osteoarthritis or hypertension. The decision to lose weight induces her to consult a doctor, who offers advice and suggests a stringent diet. In most cases of obesity it is difficult for an obese person to adhere to a stringent diet, which contains less than 5040 kJ (1200 kcals) per day, because previously she has eaten at least twice and often four times this amount of energy each day. In this she resembles a 'binge-eater'. She wants to keep to the diet but she is tempted to eat. The decision to keep to a diet becomes even harder when a severely obese person has already lost substantial weight. Every day, in every social situation, she has to make a decision, and keep to it, that she will not eat food which other people are eating freely. She knows that she should keep her weight down, for whatever reason she first chose to reduce her weight, but she finds it frustrating to do so. She begins to think about food and to plan a diet. The more she plans, the more she becomes preoccupied with food and the harder it is for her to keep to her diet. She may decide to abandon all attempts to diet, or may start binge-eating. Another choice is to seek to have some form of operation which will protect her at least partially from eating readily available food.

The main key to weight loss is the motivation to permanently alter eating behaviour. It is also evident that most obese people must have eaten more food over the years than non-obese people or they would not be so fat.

In these two respects, obesity is an eating disorder, and its correction must involve methods by which the obese person finds it 'better', psychologically and physically, to reduce weight than to remain obese. The treatment of obesity therefore requires the person to change her eating habits.

Obesity as an eating disorder

Further evidence that obesity is an eating disorder are the comments made by severely obese patients when placed on low-energy diets. Most have adverse emotional reactions. The main problems are a pre-occupation with food (65–75 per cent), irritability (60–70 per cent), nervousness (40–50 per cent), and depression (35–45 per cent). These symptoms are similar to those voiced by bulimic patients and women who have anorexia nervosa.

Obesity can be defined in several ways, some of which require complex investigations and are only practical in research. Other definitions are less complicated, and enable a person to determine if she is obese. A simple and effective method is to use the Body Mass Index (W/H^2) or BMI (for a definition see page 24). Using the BMI several groups can be identified, the last three relating to obesity (Table 12).

Generally overweight and obesity are defined as an excess of body fat, but a few very muscular men may be classified as overweight (on the BMI formula) although they have no excess of body fat. However, the BMI ratio of these men does not exceed 29, so they are not obese, by definition, although they may appear overweight. They can be differentiated from other overweight people relatively easily. When the person's weight places her in the classification of morbid obesity, medical conditions which are potentially life-threatening become more common and help is more urgently required. These grades are arbitrary to some extent. The BMI is also useful to categorize the

Table 12. Body Mass Index related to ranges of body weight

	BMI range
Emaciated	less than 15
Severely underweight	15.0–16.9
Underweight	17.0–18.9
Normal weight range	19.0–24.9
Overweight	25.0–29.9
Obese	30.0–39.9
Severely (morbidly) obese	40.0 or more

degree by which people are underweight or overweight as is shown in Table 12.

The prevalence of eating disorders in the community

The exact prevalence of eating disorders in the community is difficult to determine accurately. Most surveys are made of groups selected for the ease of surveying, such as women attending school, or are obtained by advertising in women's magazines. Women who have an eating disorder, particularly if it is severe, may be unrepresented in these surveys either because they do not want to disclose their problem or because they were absent from their place of study or work, or were being treated in hospital when the survey was made.

It is increasingly clear from a review of published studies, that women of all social classes and of many racial groups may have an eating disorder, and the older belief that bulimia nervosa and anorexia nervosa were almost exclusively found in middle-class, caucasian women is incorrect. The prevalence of obesity is more difficult to estimate, as obesity increases with age and reaches its peak prevalence in both women and men between the ages of 50 and 70.

Current information suggests that the following figures give a reasonable estimate of the prevalence of the eating disorders in women aged 15 to 30.

Anorexia nervosa: 0.5–1.0 per cent
Bulimia nervosa: 2 per cent (range 1–3 per cent)
EDNOS*:   12 per cent (range 8–23 per cent)
Obesity: 10 per cent.
*includes binge-eating disorder

The future

As our knowledge of the eating disorders increases, we hope that a range of facilities will be developed where patients can be treated by health professionals who are experienced in treating eating disorders. The choices of treatment facilities and the health professionals chosen will depend on the sufferers' individual problems and the severity of the disorder. For example, live-in/go-out (for study and work) homes could replace full in-patient treatment for some anorexia nervosa sufferers.

These matters are discussed more fully in the following chapters.

3 Why do eating disorders occur?

What made me anorexic in the first instance seems to be unimportant to what keeps me as thin as I am. I've come to the right conclusion that my anorexia is just a bad habit and a crutch for any failings I may wish to excuse myself from making.

In spite of a considerable amount of research in the past three decades no consensus has been obtained to answer the question: Why do some adolescents have an eating disorder? Five explanations have been advanced, but none of them has been proved conclusively. They are (1) the developmental and learning theory explanation; (2) the social explanation; (3) the psychological explanation; (4) the physiological explanation; and (5) the genetic explanation. These theories are not mutually exclusive and referring to more than one may give a closer explanation.

The developmental and learning theory explanation

From the earliest days of its life the quality of care a mother gives to her baby, and the love she lavishes on the baby, are related at least indirectly to the amount of fat covering its body. A chubby baby is seen by the mother and her neighbours as a well-cared-for baby. In childhood, too, the provision of substantial amounts of food, often rich in refined carbohydrates and fat, is seen as a way of showing love for children, as well as ensuring that they are adequately nourished. In our culture, which has an abundance of food, children learn to increase progressively the amount of food they eat, and often increase the quantity of energy they ingest beyond that needed for growth, body functions, and the demands of exercise. In the three years before puberty, a biological spurt of growth occurs, and the food intake is increased still further.

Studies have shown that in boys the energy requirements for growth, and the spurt in growth, occur at about the age of 15; and because boys increase their muscle mass after this age, additional energy continues to be needed. The growth spurt in girls occurs between the ages of 12 and 14, earlier than that of boys, and the girl's energy requirements peak over the same period. After her first menstrual period the girl's energy requirements have fallen considerably, as girls do not increase their muscle mass like boys. Most girls reduce their food intake or take more exercise so that their weight only increases slowly, and some girls seem able to eat as they wish without becoming overweight or obese. A few girls continue to eat the amount of food they have become accustomed to during the period of growth in early adolescence and put on weight, becoming overweight or obese.

In the year after menarche the young woman becomes increasingly aware of her body weight; she learns that she can control weight gain by eating sensibly, changing her eating patterns, dieting, or by using other measures which will help her to stop her absorbing the food she eats (see Chapter 1 figs 3,4).

On the other hand, some adolescents may reject the need to control their weight and may enjoy eating, while limiting the amount of energy expended in exercise. Inevitably this will lead to obesity. Some of the adolescents who diet and control their weight successfully may become so concerned about food and about weight control that their eating behaviour escapes from what is considered 'normal', and they decide to pursue thinness—becoming anorexia nervosa victims. Some of those who diet unsuccessfully either develop bulimia nervosa or become obese. Some adolescent women who present with an eating disorder have mothers, fathers, and sisters who are vocally critical of their daughter's appearance and weight. Mothers and older sisters may also have experienced difficulties adjusting to the weight challenge following menarche and a few may have developed an eating disorder.

Onset of severe weight loss can also follow a period of sensible dieting with realistic weight loss or, in some of the younger patients,

Case history: Vera

Vera first became concerned about her weight when she was aged 14, nearly 12 months after her first monstrual period, and started dieting. However her preoccupation with food caused her to gain weight in spite of the diet she had chosen. She was teased about her body by her friends and in an attempt to lose weight effectively began taking large quantities of laxatives when she was 16. Soon after she began to abuse laxatives. Her menstrual periods ceased. The next year, a series of family problems and her continued concern about her body image induced her to adhere to a weight-reducing diet (5040 kJ (1200 kcal) a day) with resultant weight loss. By the age of 18 her weight had stabilized at a level she found acceptable (BMI 21) and has maintained this weight, with fluctuations of 1–3 kg (2.2–6.6 lbs), for the past five years.

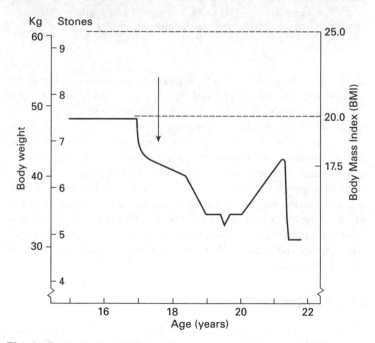

Fig. 9. Robin started dieting at the age of 14. By the age of 17 she had developed anorexia nervosa (A) and this has persisted in spite of treatment since that date.

Case history: Kate

Kate began to 'watch her weight' when she was at boarding school, as did many of her contemporaries. However, the nature of the food and the discipline imposed on the students limited her ability to control her weight. She left school at 18, having graduated from high school, and became increasingly conscious of her weight. She decided that she wanted to lose weight by 'avoiding eating rubbish'. She was now at university, and began binge-eating, interspersing this with stringent dieting, which resulted in wide swings of weight. In an attempt to control her weight gain, at the age of 19 she began to self-induce vomiting and abused both laxatives and diuretics. This behaviour coincided with a decision to leave university and to move to another city to take up fashion modelling. To some extent her behaviour controlled the swings in her weight, but she continued to have episodes of binge-eating, although these became less frequent, but it was not until she was aged 24 that she achieved a body weight below a BMI of 19. She has since stabilized at a BMI of 18.5 by keeping to a strict eating plan, and she no longer uses laxatives and diuretics.

it appears to occur immediately, with no prior unsuccessful or realistic attempts. On the other hand, the young woman may reject the need to be or to become thin and may continue eating the quantity of food she has learned to eat and enjoys eating. If she was fat during early adolescence, the degree of obesity will increase. Obesity occurs in some families, and may be due to the family having a continuing fantasy that 'our family have always had healthy appetites and have been large people'. A child brought up in such a family is comfortable over-eating and becoming obese because she can share an identity with the other members of her family. She has no need to change her eating patterns in adolescence to conform with prevailing fashions because the strong influence of her family outweighs those of prevailing fashion.

The social explanation

In Western culture two contrasting messages about food and eating are offered by society, and particularly by the media. The first message is that a slim woman is successful, attractive, healthy, happy, fit, and popular. Most teenagers believe that being slim will help them to be chosen for a good job, find a boy-friend, be popular with their peers, be and look fit and healthy, and get on well with their family (provided that most of the family is not overweight or obese). To become slim, with all that this implies, is deemed to be a major pursuit of many women. The second message is that eating is a pleasurable activity which meets many needs, in addition to relieving hunger, and women have a right to have these needs met. In women's magazines these two contrasting messages tend to appear inextricably mixed. In nearly every issue the magazines publish 'exciting' new diets which 'guarantee weight loss with minimum discomfort or motivation'—and these diets are often followed by recipes for, and superb photographs of, luscious cakes and foods with rich sauces. It is difficult to watch television without being confronted by an advertisement for a substitute low-energy food alternating with a fast-food advertisement, or its equivalent. The social (and usually

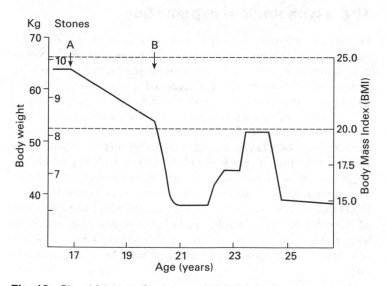

Fig. 10. Cheryl felt herself to be overweight when she was aged 17 and started dieting. At that time her BMI was 24 (A). The dieting resulted in a slow weight loss until the age of 20, when she broke up with her boy-friend and had a sudden weight loss, leading to a diagnosis of anorexia nervosa (B).

family) pressures are also contradictory: you must eat everything other people give you but you must not get fat.

The provision of food is seen in our culture as a major sign of caring; and sharing food at a meal is seen as one of the prime social contacts. These cultural imperatives place a burden on a parent to provide abundant quantities of food, and on her loving daughter or son to eat that food. It is not surprising that in the face of the psychological bombardment of two contradictory messages, most young women diet. Some develop bulimia nervosa. Others become preoccupied with food and the avoidance of weight gain, developing bulimia or anorexia nervosa. Some decide that dieting is too disturbing to their way of life and return to eating more food than they require, becoming obese. These women may also find obesity protective against acceding to current social attitudes to sexuality, which they fear. Hidden in a fat body, they give the message that they are not attractive and do not want to form a sexual relationship.

The psychological explanation

Because eating is such a basic instinct it has been postulated that those people who suffer from an eating disorder have an identifiable personality, being more obsessional or neurotic than normal eaters. The *Oxford textbook of psychiatry* defines personality as 'enduring qualities of an individual shown in his or her ways of behaving in a wide variety of circumstances'. Some studies, using personality questionnaires, suggest that some women suffering from anorexia nervosa are indeed more 'neurotic' or 'obsessional', have 'self-loathing' and lower self-esteem than women whose weight is in the 'desirable range'. The studies also suggest that those women who have lost weight by dieting and excessive exercise are more introverted, more anxious, and more dependent than women whose weight is normal or women with anorexia nervosa who use self-induced vomiting and purgation as methods of losing weight. No distinctive personality profiles are available for women who have bulimia nervosa or for obese women. Most have poor self-esteem.

The *Oxford textbook of psychiatry* defines an abnormal personality as occurring 'when the individual suffers from his own personality or when other people suffer from it'. The American Psychiatric Association defines a 'personality disorder' as being present when 'the constellation of behaviours or traits causes either significant impairment in social or occupational functioning or subjective distress'. Could it be that patients with eating disorders have an abnormal personality or a personality disorder?

The American Psychiatric Association has suggested a further subgroup of personality disorder which they term a 'borderline personality disorder'. For this diagnosis to be made, the person must have at least five of the following eight features: unstable relationships; impulsive behaviour that is harmful to the person (including spending, sex, substance use, shop-lifting, reckless driving, and binge-eating); variable moods; undue anger or lack of control of anger; recurrent suicidal threats or behaviour; uncertainty about personal identity; persistent feelings of boredom; and frantic efforts to avoid real or imagined abandonment. This definition may cause diagnostic problems. For example, does a young male, living in a slum neighbourhood, who shop-lifts, steals cars for joy-riding, has undue anger and is often in fights, has an unstable relationship and persistent feelings of boredom, have a personality disorder when, in his culture, these behaviours are so common that they are considered normal? This suggests that a major problem in accepting the concept of a borderline personality disorder is that it is imprecise and may depend on environmental and socio-cultural influences.

Women who are in the usual age-group for diagnosis of an eating disorder may have several of the features required for the diagnosis of a borderline personality disorder. When people recover from an eating disorder only a few have a personality disorder, most do not.

However, in women with an eating disorder, some of the features are due to the biochemical and psychological changes (discussed later in this chapter) resulting from the eating disorder—for example, variable moods and feelings of chronic boredom. If they are added to another of the features needed to make a diagnosis of a borderline personality disorder, the total may appear to clinch the diagnosis, whilst in reality, the woman does not have a personality disorder. She may have a temporary change in her personality soon after the onset of the eating disorder, or episodically during the disorder. Such a change has been reported frequently by the family or by people with whom the woman lives.

Until a more precise definition of personality disorder has been made, all that can be said is that a woman may have both an eating disorder and a personality disorder, but not that most people who have an eating disorder have a personality disorder. Further problems about accepting a psychological explanation for the eating disorder are, first, that many women who have anorexia nervosa or bulimia nervosa have been found, after careful testing, to have a 'normal' personality and second, the personality scores of normal people and those who suffer from eating disorders overlap considerably. This may mean that the tests are too crude to identify a personality problem, or that the psychological explanation has no foundation.

Other psychological explanations have been suggested, one of which is the concept that some obese women use eating as a substitute for love. A person who feels lonely, empty, and unloved unless she has constant company may eat to compensate. The emptiness of her life is soothed if she takes food to fill her empty stomach. The more she eats the more complete and full (or fulfilled) she feels. Food, and particularly beverages such as milk or beer, become mainstays of her life, suppressing lack of self-esteem and providing satisfaction. As she becomes increasingly obese she develops a need to remain obese and so avoid the resurgence of her feeling of inadequacy.

Furthermore, according to the personality defect theory, some women suffering from anorexia nervosa have a fear of 'growing up' and of becoming physically and sexually mature. By avoiding eating, the woman's body contours become those of a prepubertal child, her menstrual periods either do not start or cease, she is able to withdraw from the social occasions which make her ill at ease and anxious, and is able to deny her sexuality. This explanation may apply to a few anorexia nervosa patients, but in most cases of eating disorders the concept does not apply.

From this it follows that although psychological factors may be involved in explaining why individual patients who have an eating disorder persist with their eating behaviour, no single psychological explanation is available.

The physiological explanation

Recent research has shown that many people who embark on a strict diet feel 'flat and down in mood'. These people have been found to have low levels of tryptophan in their blood. After eating food, particularly foods with a high carbohydrate content, the level of tryptophan in the blood is raised. The increase is due to a release of insulin following the absorption of the food, which increases the ratio of tryptophan to other amino acids.

The raised circulating level of tryptophan permits it to cross from the blood into the brain where it stimulates the production of serotonin (5-hydroxytryptamine or 5HT). The raised brain level of serotonin decreases the person's appetite and improves the person's mood.

Recently, in a double-blind, placebo-controlled study we gave tryptophan in a high dose of 3 g a day and vitamin B_6 in a dose of 50 mg a day (which is said to improve the uptake of tryptophan into the brain) to 11 women being treated for bulimia nervosa. The drug and the placebo were in identical capsules and neither we nor the patients knew which was being taken. Each woman filled in a Mood and Behaviour Questionnaire each night just before going to bed.

When the results were analysed we found that during the time that the women were taking tryptophan, they reported an improvement in mood, less binge-eating, less overeating, and less 'picking behaviour'. In addition, when they did binge-eat the amount of food eaten was reduced. However the changes in binge-eating were small, which suggests that the tryptophan theory does not in itself fully explain why people binge-eat (Table 13).

Table 13. Tryptophan and pyridoxine in the treatment of bulimia nervosa (11 women studied in a randomized, crossover, double-blind trial)

	Average daily scores*	
	Women taking tryptophan	**Women taking placebo**
Total mood score	43.3	47.3
Binge-earing	0.32	0.52
Overeating	0.59	0.85
'Picking'	0.30	0.52
Eating out of control	0.55	0.73
Amount eaten in binge	0.41	0.78

* The lower the average daily score the more improvement shown

Many other factors have now been discovered that affect the messenger substances (neurotransmitters), serotonin and noradrenaline in the brain. One of these is a hormone called leptin that is produced by the adipose (fat) cells of the body. Leptin appears to regulate appetite by its action on the part of the brain called the hypothalamus. Leptin levels are very high in the blood of obese people as they have more fat in the cells of the body. These high leptin levels in the blood going to the brain should cause the release of serotonin and noradrenaline that result in feelings of satiation, fullness, and a lack of appetite.

For some reason obese people appear to be relatively insensitive to leptin. The sufferer of chronic obesity has a problem preventing weight gain; most can lose weight but cannot stop it returning. It is likely that leptin is important in this apparent failure of obese people to be able to 'reset' their body weight at a lower weight after weight loss. Genetic influences may explain the insensitivity of the brain to leptin or the receptors in the brain may adapt and become less affected by high levels of leptin after a long period of time. Some obese people may choose to ignore the feelings of satiation and lack of appetite and continue to eat more food than they require or they may choose to eat for other reasons including anxiety and sometimes depression.

People with normal weight bulimia nervosa may have a normal response to the raised levels of leptin and the other messages from the blood, gut, hormones, and nerves after eating. They may be constantly dieting to try to attain a body weight that is below their genetically determined 'set point'. There are a variety of chemicals in the brain called neuropeptides that stimulate and decrease appetite. When bulimia nervosa sufferers try to restrict their food intake they receive messages to eat; neuroepeptide Y is the most powerful substance that drives the person to eat. In a binge a large amount of food is eaten rapidly and it is not until hours later that the body can integrate all the information and respond by decreasing the urge to eat. During this time eating may have continued, albeit with decreased fervour, or additional binges may have occurred. Women who do not induce vomiting find the drive to binge-eat is less following an episode or day of binge-eating and feel that they can again diet and exercise, but after 2 days of restricted eating they again have an overwhelming urge to binge-eat. Why bulimia nervosa sufferers feel they cannot resist the powerful urge to eat is unknown. It is possible that they become sensitised to one or more of the neuropeptides that drive people to eat or that they crave feelings of well-being, such as the improved mood and lack of appetite provided by increased brain levels of serotonin after eating. The conflicting and confusing messages the body receives when bulimics induce vomiting may take many years to be fully understood.

Anorexia nervosa is more difficult to fit into the tryptophan/serotonin theory. Anorexia nervosa patients initially deny themselves eating an adequate amount of food and do not respond to the 'messages' to eat more food and feel better. If they continue to eat inadequate amounts of food for their bodily functions over a period of time, one hypothesis suggests that an increase in opioid activity occurs in their brains. This leads to an elevation of the person's mood and causes the person to continue restricting food because it makes her feel 'good'. As time passes, the elevation of mood can only be maintained by reducing the food intake further, and 'addiction' to increased brain opioids may be inevitable if withdrawal symptoms are to be avoided.

Anorexia nervosa patients who have episodes of breaking their strict diet and who have small eating binges do not reach such low weights and find it easier to gain weight than women whose eating behaviour is restrictive. The theory could explain this finding by suggesting that these women do not become so 'addicted' to high brain opioid levels and can respond, at least episodically, to the need to eat.

Exercise is also thought to cause the release of opioids into the brain and the more strenuous the exercise the greater the opioid release. The need for some people to increase the amount of exercise that they undertake can be explained by their need to maintain the release of brain opioids.

Many women who have anorexia nervosa exercise excessively when at low body weight and during weight loss, or during and after refeeding. This behaviour may be explained by a brain opioid 'addiction'.

These theories await further clarification. If they are correct, anorexia nervosa patients may be trying to stimulate their mood and they equate euphoria with a decreased food intake. Bulimia nervosa patients and some obese patients eat because the food induces the release of brain serotonin which may improve their mood to help them relax, which they equate with increased food intake.

The genetic explanation

The question of whether a defective gene is the cause of the eating disorder is currently being investigated. Information gathered suggests that in a *few* sufferers a possible genetic defect may be involved, particularly involving overweight and obese people. For most sufferers, however, no such cause can be found. Despite this we know that genes do play a part in the development of anorexia nervosa, bulimia nervosa, EDNOS, and obesity. These disorders are more common in identical (monozygotic) twins compared with non-identical twins (dizygotic) and more common in siblings and families when compared to the population. Some members of a family develop different eating disorders, for example, one sister may be 'bulimic' and the other 'anorexic'.

It may be easier to understand the failure to find a defective gene if you consider that people with the genetic potential will only develop an eating disorder if certain events take place, that is, the events allow the genes to express themselves. A highly respected researcher into the genetics of mental illness, called Kendler, suggests that society's current preoccupation with thinness and body image has allowed more people who carry the genes for anorexia nervosa and bulimia nervosa to develop the disorder. Fifty years ago, before society emphasized a slim body shape and weight as desirable, these people may not have suffered from an eating disorder. Our recent work suggests being female and attaining menarche may also be needed to allow young women with 'at risk' genes to develop an eating disorder. Multiple environmental, personality, and physiological factors may also be involved.

The combined explanation

No single explanation is sufficient to explain why eating disorders occur. The genetic explanation accounts for only a few sufferers. The developmental and learning theory explanation and the social explanation may answer the question of why eating disorders are more likely to occur in women and the onset is more likely to occur in the late teens or in the early 20s; but not why only some women develop an eating disorder, or why the eating disorder persists for many years in only a few women. Perhaps the psychological or physiological explanations may help to explain this. A model to show the combined explanation is given in Fig. 11. This multidiscipline concept was adapted from a model proposed for the assessment and prediction of suicide by Maris, Bergman, and Maltsberger in 1992.

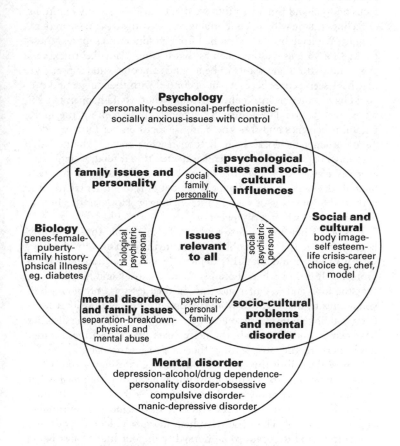

Fig. 11. A multidiscipline explanation for the development of eating disorders

What is an eating disorder? A sufferer's view

One of our patients wrote this letter to her parents.

Dear Mum and Dad,

I thought that I would write this letter in an attempt to try and explain what an eating disorder actually is. From talking to you about it on various occasions I have come to realize that both of you still view an eating disorder as a diet. The truth of the matter is that we focus on food and weight so that we don't have to feel any emotions or feelings that may be uncomfortable, such as anger, sadness, anxiety, or guilt. We have been conditioned from childhood to suppress these feelings for various reasons, such as that it is not 'ladylike' to express them and that no one wants to be around someone who is upset. We may have seen people become out of control with their anger and this could have scared us into believing that's what would happen to us if we became angry. The longer we suppress these feelings the more painful it becomes and thus the more we focus on our food in a desperate attempt to block them. It soon reaches a stage when all the emotions that we feel are indeed connected to our food, weight, and shape. We grow to believe that we are void of all feelings. Inside us a big hole develops and in attempt to get out of it we either try to fill it with food by bingeing or we try to starve it away. However this hole is bottomless and will not disappear.

It is only when we come to a place like this clinic that we slowly begin to realize that our problem is not anything to do with the food we eat or avoid and that this is just a symptom of our underlying problems. It is only when these issues are discussed and help is given that the food and weight issues can become less of a problem.when you are ready, that you can work through all the emotions that have been building up inside of you over the years that the eating disorder has been around. Obviously the more years that the eating disorder has been there, the more feelings there are to get through.

I know that all of this must sound pretty confusing to you. I feel that the most important thing for you to remember is that *food* is not the problem. Most anorexics do not set out with the aim of losing weight to any extent. However once it has begun it is extremely difficult to control. Then you need help in order to stop the destructive pattern and to regain some normality in your life. So just being taught to eat properly does not mean that you can simply eat normally when you leave here.

I hope that this has helped a bit to explain what an eating disorder is. It is a bit confusing to us, so I can imagine that to non-sufferers a lot of the behaviours would be incomprehensible. Why would someone starve themselves to a near death? Why can't they start to eat when they look like a skeleton? Why don't they get to see how thin they are? I think most anorexics do realize that they are thin when they are badly underweight, but they still feel fat and big. That never changes.

Anyway that is about all I can say about what I see an eating disorder as being about. It is caused for a variety of reasons. Often it is not just one event but a chain of events that builds up the stress that has been suppressed.

The writer then goes on to explain about her personal problems, which, to preserve her anonymity, we will omit.

Preventing the onset of an eating disorder

Most patients suffering from anorexia nervosa present for help in early adolescence. Most patients with bulimia nervosa present in late adolescence or in their early twenties. Obese patients tend to present in their late twenties or later.

Eating disorder sufferers usually have had the disorder for several years before seeking help and many never seek help. In the case of anorexia nervosa and bulimia nervosa the disorder is preceded in most cases by episodes of dieting and other weight-losing behaviours because the adolescent believes that she is too fat. Between the episodes of dieting, she may go on eating-binges. These behaviours are no different from over 70 per cent of adolescent girls, except they are more extreme and the girl appears to have lost control of her eating behaviours.

Is there any strategy which would help the few who develop an eating disorder avoiding this outcome, or at least presenting early in the disorder when, with treatment, the outcome is better? Several interventions have been tried but none has been successful. One untested intervention which might help is for magazines designed for teenagers to provide accurate information about the various eating disorders, rather than the sensational stories which are currently published, so that some affected teenagers might seek help earlier.

Suitable articles might include stories about teenage women who have a variety of shapes and body weights. It is possible that such articles might encourage young women to feel more comfortable with their appearance. Care must be taken that this approach does not inadvertantly make some women feel worse about themselves.

To a small extent these changes in emphasis are beginning to appear. Magazines, read by women, now print stories about women of different ethnic backgrounds and about women who are athletic 'heros'. Other articles might be written which would help young women feel good about themselves—in other words increase their self-esteem—de-emphasizing that physical appearance is the most important way a person is judged.

School programmes are also being developed to improve the self-esteem of young teenagers. Again these de-emphasize physical appearance and help young women to have a more realistic perception of their body image.

4

Eating disorders and sexuality

Often I used to go out and eat for my sensual sexual experience of the day. I actually would be turned on by it.

Coming to terms with one's sexuality is a major challenge facing adolescents. It appears that many women who have an eating disorder perceive an association between eating and sexuality. The sexual knowledge, attitudes, and behaviour of women with eating disorders covers a broad spectrum. This is not surprising as many are over-concerned about their body image and their relationships with others. In addition sexual feelings and lubrication of the vagina during sexual arousal are decreased when women lose weight. This is caused by a decrease in the same hormones that are associated with the disturbance in menstruation (see page 156). We have found that there is an association between the eating behaviour and sexual behaviour of the women we have studied, and have identified four categories of sexual behaviour: sexuality denied; unsure of sexuality; sexually passive; and sexually active.

Sexuality denied

The woman avoids challenge to her sexuality and suppresses her sexual feelings. She has negative attitudes to puberty, menstruation, masturbation, and sexual intercourse. These attitudes may be aggravated by her lack of knowledge of her genital anatomy, of menstruation, of contraception, and of sexual behaviour. She avoids reading about sexuality and is rigid and obsessional in her attitudes to life. She avoids looking at her body in a mirror, and does not touch her genitals. She uses external sanitary pads for menstrual protection and has never attempted to use tampons. Most of the women in this group have long periods of amenorrhoea, no sexual experience, and neither masturbate nor date. They become embarrassed if a discussion relates to sex, but often wish that they had a close companion. These women lose weight exclusively by strict dieting and exercise, and often are very emaciated.

Case history: Clarissa

Clarissa is aged 28, is an only child, and is a highly intelligent, personable, neatly dressed woman, but rather obsessional and anxious. She finds it difficult to relate socially. She learned about menstruation when she was 13 from her mother, who was embarrassed and not very informative. Six months later she had her first menstrual period. She was ashamed and embarrassed about menstruating, and described her periods as 'messy', 'dirty', 'disgusting', and 'inconvenient'. She was unable to touch herself 'down there', and used sanitary pads, which she continues to use. She feels unable to use tampons. She received no information about sexuality or sexual intercourse from her mother, and felt unable to ask anyone else because of her shyness. She has avoided reading any books about sexuality, and says that 'there is no point because I wouldn't remember any of the information'.

At the age of 20 she had her first relationship, but it broke up after two years because she believed that the man was 'making demands on her', and because she couldn't cope with his desire for sex. She has since avoided any physical contact with a man. She finds it difficult to say words describing sexual functions, and found kissing 'disgusting' although she permitted her boyfriend to kiss her occasionally. The idea of sexual intercourse revolts her, particularly as she would be forced to look at and touch the man's genitals. She has a dread of exposing her body and of looking at her breasts, abdomen, or thighs in a mirror.

She began dieting soon after her relationship ended. Her object in dieting was to reduce the size of her breasts (which she saw as large and ugly although her boyfriend had complimented her on their shape) and to take weight off her abdomen. By the age of 23 she was considerably underweight and her menstrual periods had ceased. She says that she is pleased about this as she hated menstruating and she uses her thinness to avoid social situations and sexual challenges. She is 'up-tight' and fastidious in her appearance and, at work, her employer refers to her as 'a most excellent secretary'.

Case history: Clarissa (continued)

In the past five years she has had episodes of dramatic weight loss, due to stringent dieting alone, which have required admission to hospital for refeeding. She has never induced vomiting, having a fear of its effects, nor does she abuse laxatives or diuretics. Her rigid dieting and her sexual attitudes appear to be part of a constant preoccupation with 'self control' and a desire for perfection. She is not sure what masturbation is and would never attempt it. She denies any sexual feelings and says she has never accepted that she 'could have a libido'. However, the thought that she might be a lesbian causes her to avoid female company. She is 'disgusted' by homosexuality. She is often lonely and wishes for a male or female companion, but avoids making friends, believing herself unable to cope with an intimacy that could lead to a sexual challenge. Amenorrhoea has been 'a relief' which she hopes will continue.

Unsure of sexuality

These women appear to use their eating behaviour to delay sexual encounters until they feel that they are ready for them. The woman tends to find it difficult to form a warm, mature relationship, although she may marry, when she tends to be dependent on her husband. She is anxious to conform and has conflicts about her sexual feelings and her sexual behaviour, always trying to be what she believes is 'normal'. She is shy. She may masturbate occasionally but worries because it may not be 'right' to masturbate. If she is given reassurance that her sexual behaviour is 'normal' she can begin to enjoy it. She is shy, and, although she may look at her naked body in a mirror, does not feel comfortable when doing it. She is also shy about menstrual protection and prefers sanitary pads to tampons, as she finds the latter 'difficult' to insert. Her anxiety about vaginal insertion extends to sexual intercourse, which usually first takes place at an older age than average. She believes that she is not easily aroused, but sometimes reaches orgasm either by clitoral stimulation or during sexual intercourse.

Women in this group lose weight predominantly by dieting and exercising. If they decide to use laxatives or diuretics, they only take small quantities for short periods of time. Usually they have anorexia nervosa but may be obese.

Case history: Samantha

Samantha is aged 26 and is an attractive 'elfin' woman who is dependent on others and needs continual reassurance and approval about her relationship with both sexes. She learnt about menstruation and sexuality from a book (given to her by her mother) when she was 12 years old. She went to a boarding school run by nuns, and was worried when her menstrual periods failed to start, as all the other girls in her class were menstruating. She became increasingly anxious and apprehensive about starting to menstruate, and was embarrassed when, at the age of 15, her first menstrual period began during a dancing class. Sex education was not provided at school, but she was told that it was wrong and unhealthy to masturbate. When she tried masturbation she felt guilty and ashamed and did not repeat the experience. During her last two years at school, she dieted, unsuccessfully, with school friends, and her weight increased slightly, although it stayed within the 'desirable' range. She was self-conscious about the small size of her breasts, and the fact that whilst her school friends *needed* bras she just *wore* one.

She left school and entered university, where she began dieting. This resulted in weight loss and her menstrual periods ceased, which pleased her, saying she 'felt lucky they had stopped because she hated them'. Towards the end of the first year in university, she formed a relationship with another student. She knew herself to be sexually ignorant and although her ignorance worried her she did not seek any sexual information. She permitted nothing more than kissing in the relationship. The relationship lasted two months, and after it ended she continued to diet strictly and lose weight. When she was 20 she met her future husband. By this time she was very thin. During their four year courtship she limited sexual contact to kissing, and occasional breast stimulation, although she did not enjoy this because of the small size of her breasts. Before the marriage at the age of 24, she visited her family doctor who prescribed oral contraception. She tried to use a tampon during the first episode of withdrawn bleeding but reverted to pads as 'it was difficult and uncomfortable to put the thing in'. At marriage she was emaciated and fulfilled the criteria for anorexia nervosa. She had a romantic opinion about marriage and believed that once married she would 'blossom'. The first attempt at sexual intercourse was a 'dismal failure', which disillusioned her. Subsequent intercourse has often been painful and the couple tend to avoid sex. She alternates between blaming herself and her husband who she says is 'undersexed'. She has never discussed sex with him

Case history: Samantha (continued)
because of embarrassment and the belief that she is 'frigid'. When they have sexual intercourse, she tells him she enjoys it, and has fantasies of responding more if they could vary positions during sexual intercourse, but feels too inhibited to suggest the idea. She has never had an orgasm during sexual intercourse, but says she can sometimes reach orgasm if her husband stimulates her clitoris. Her husband enjoys swimming but she refuses to go with him as she thinks she is too thin and is embarrassed about her small breasts. At times she wishes she was 'soft and cuddly' like most women.

Sexually passive

Women in this group (which includes those who have anorexia nervosa, bulimia, or who are obese) also appear to use their eating disorder to avoid having to make a sexual commitment until they want to. The woman's eating behaviour offers her a chance to place an 'intermittent moratorium' on her sexual activity. She experiences wide swings in weight, binge-eating alternating with periods of fasting or strict dieting. If she is bulimic, she rarely reaches a low weight and if she does she maintains the low weight only for a short period of time, before binge-eating and gaining weight. Between underweight and overweight episodes, women in this group become involved in sexual relationships, but are unresponsive, denying that they enjoy their experiences. Because they do not wish for a commitment they tend to choose partners who are married, and with whom a long-term relationship is not possible. In the relationship they prefer to cuddle and be held, and accept sexual intercourse to achieve this rather than because they enjoy the experience. They are able to touch their genitals and use tampons for menstrual protection, but their ability to look at their body depends on their weight at the time.

Case history: Harriet
Harriet, who is aged 25, is an attractive, overweight young woman who desperately wanted to lose weight in order to attract a boyfriend and to 'live a normal life'. Before she had menstruated (when she was 13 years old) her mother had told her about menstruation and she had been

Case history: Harriet (continued)

shown a film at school. For two years she suffered from pain and vomiting with her menstrual periods and wished to be rid of them. She used pads until changing to tampons when she was 18. At the age of 14 she had a brief lesbian relationship at school but felt it 'did nothing' for her. When she was 16, she decided to 'stop eating rubbish' and reduced her weight by dieting. At the age of 17 she applied for and was accepted for a teachers' training course and began alternating between binge-eating and stringent dieting. In addition she abused laxatives. During the course and subsequently when teaching in primary school the eating behaviour caused at least five rapid swings in weight. She wanted to lose weight from her 'bottom, stomach, and thighs' and would look at her body in a mirror when her weight was low, but avoided looking when she was 'fat'. She dressed to camouflage her body when she was obese but not when she was thin. Over a three-month period her weight could vary from 44 kg (97 lbs, 6st 13 lbs; BMI 19) to 57 kg (126 lbs, 9 st; BMI 25).

Throughout the six years her menstrual pattern was quite irregular and she did not bother to record when she menstruated. She considered sex 'normal' and wished to lose her virginity 'as quickly as possible', in order to 'satisfy curiosity', 'to rebel against' her parents, and to achieve 'maturity'. She believed sexual intercourse was necessary to attract and keep a boyfriend. At the age of 18 she had intercourse six weeks after meeting her first boyfriend. She described her first experience of penetration as 'fantastic because of the pain'. Later experiences were not painful but 'never satisfying'. During the 12 months of her first sexual relationship her weight fluctuated within the normal range. She used the contraceptive pill throughout the relationship. She ended the relationship because of recurrence of bulimia and consequent weight increase. Renewed dieting lowered her weight but when she began binge-eating her weight continued to rise. Her second sexual contact was during a five-month stabilization of weight. She had hoped to gain a friend by agreeing to have sexual intercourse but felt obliged to terminate the relationship after renewed binge-eating. Desperation with weight gain culminated in a suicide attempt by an overdose of sleeping tablets. She has 'never really enjoyed' orogenital sex and prefers to be the recipient. She will only use a passive, supine position for sexual intercourse. She feels guilty about masturbating and states that she has turned to binge-eating as a 'substitute'. After the commencement of treatment and an initial weight reduction she maintained her weight within the normal range for 10 months during which time she resumed

Case history: Harriet (continued)
sexual activity with two older, married men which she enjoyed but found sexually unrewarding. She stopped abusing laxatives and the frequency of her eating binges was reduced from weekly to monthly episodes. The relationships were terminated during a brief episode of bulimic behaviour with a resultant rise in weight of 4 kg (9 lbs). Her weight has subsequently been stable within the normal range for six months and sexual activity has resumed.

Sexually assertive

Women in this group mirror their eating behaviour, which consists of binge-eating followed by episodes of self-induced vomiting and laxative abuse, with their sexual behaviour. They are unable to form a long-term relationship and have frequent casual sexual encounters. They usually have had their first sexual experience at an early age; they masturbate and have oral sex, but are rather negative about both of these. They talk about sex freely and have no anxiety about being naked, either when alone or with others. They tend to be histrionic, and socially active, but underlying this is a feeling of loneliness.

Case history: Brenda
Brenda is an attractive well-groomed blonde of 24 who has a rather theatrical manner. She is preoccupied with sex and likes talking and reading about it. However, she is preoccupied by doubts about her sexuality. She says she only feels feminine when her stomach is completely empty. Her mother discussed sex and masturbation with her before she went to boarding school at 12 years of age. She and a girlfriend would often explore and embrace each other in bed. She started menstruating when she was 14, which she described as 'unpleasant and a nuisance'; and it was associated with cramps requiring bed rest. She has continued to feel that her menstrual periods are 'hateful' and wishes she could 'do away with them'. For the first two menstrual cycles she used external pads and has since used tampons exclusively. She felt 'pressurized' into first intercourse at age 15 and found penetration painful and unpleasant. Subsequently she has enjoyed intercourse at times, including 'rough' intercourse. She sometimes reaches orgasm. She regrets having had sex outside marriage and wishes she could have been a 'virgin

Case history: Brenda (continued)

bride'. She has had many casual sexual partners since the age of 15. Following a 'pregnancy scare' at age 17, she developed an increased fear of pregnancy, dreading changes in body shape and the pain of childbirth, but did not use contraceptives. At age 18 she became more conscious of her weight, and dieted by avoiding 'rubbish foods'. She became engaged when she was 19, but decided she didn't really like her fiancé, and broke off the relationship. When the man married her closest girlfriend she was deeply upset and decided to move to another city where she could 'start again'. Her progress there was a disaster at first. She began binge-eating and because her weight increased she began to self-induce vomiting, and abused laxatives. She found it impossible to keep to a diet and began to drink alcohol to excess. She was very social, hated being alone, and said that on her 'good days she was the life of the party'. Increased vomiting and purging led to a steady decrease in her weight. At the lower weight she became intensely preoccupied, almost narcissistic, about her appearance and the size of her abdomen, her hips, and her thighs. Because of her appearance she obtained a job as a cosmetic representative which she enjoyed. She had multiple sexual relationships and began taking the pill. When taking oral contraceptives her menstrual periods became scanty, which pleased her. By the age of 24 her preoccupation with her body and her weight increased and she started dieting strictly, induced vomiting, and abused laxatives with the result that her body weight fell and she became emaciated. Her menstrual periods ceased when her weight was low, but she continued with multiple sexual relationships, which often involved oral and anal sex, although the latter revolted her. She says that she 'craves orgasm' and tries to get it any way she can, masturbating in the absence of other outlets. She has now been binge-eating and vomiting for five years. She has frequent invitations to parties and frequents bars and restaurants. She avoids eating before going out and prefers to wear loose fitting clothes. After returning home she induces vomiting. She feels she is most likely to vomit in a situation where she fears both sexual challenge and a temptation to 'over-eat'.

Physical and sexual abuse

The possibility that childhood physical or sexual abuse may be a factor in the development of an eating disorder has been investigated in recent years. A study of the literature indicates that about 30 per cent of eating-disorder patients will reveal that they were abused sexually in childhood, although in the majority of cases the abuse occurred only once or twice. The incidence of childhood sexual abuse among patients with eating disorders is no higher than that found among patients suffering from other psychiatric disorders. It is higher, however, than the rate of 10 to 20 per cent reported among people in the community who have no medical or psychiatric disorder.

This suggests that childhood sexual abuse may adversely affect how certain women cope with problems when they become adult, and may result in an eating disorder. Recent research suggests that women who have been abused take longer to respond to treatment and are more likely to require admission to hospital. A study in the USA found that bulimic women were more likely to have experienced sexual abuse as a child than women who suffered from a food restricting disorder. Sexual abuse as an adolescent or adult would be expected to be more common among bulimic women as they are more sexually active and more at risk because of their sexual activity or women suffering from a mixed disorder such as EDNOS.

More investigation is required to determine the relevance of childhood physical and sexual abuse in the development of an eating disorder.

Catriona describes her experiences:

I recount the following events of my childhood and the ongoing results that those events have had on my life: anxiety and an atypical eating disorder.

I can recall my father would leave home early in the morning and return home at night usually drunk, and often angry, which generally led to violent verbal and physical arguments. The arguments were not necessarily precipitated by anything that my mother or my sister had said, but I would take charge of the situation because I believed that, being Dad's favourite, I could avoid the potentially violent situation that might occur. I did not feel that it was a privilege to be the favourite. It was in fact a dreadful burden.

Dad would usually arrive home around the time of the evening meal. Mum had been trying to coax my sister into eating something from her plate instead of wanting to put everything onto a sandwich. She was a poor eater and there was a constant argument between my mother and sister during meal times. I was always praised for eating everything put in front of me. I wanted to be a 'good' daughter for my mother, because I believed it would make her life happier. During meal times, I recall being incredibly anxious waiting for my father to knock on the front door. If the knock was loud and hard, then we knew he would be angry. I would then move into control mode. I would take charge of the situation, always telling my mother not to say anything that might provoke my father's anger. I felt a tremendous burden of having to control my father's violence and anger. I would always put myself between Mum and my sister when he would threaten them, both physically and verbally. I would talk quietly and calmly; sometimes it would calm him, other times it would not. He would go into a rage and then start hitting Mum. On these occasions, we would usually have to leave the house and run to the next-door neighbours. I can recall the police being called and my mother being told that she would have to press charges against my father, otherwise they could do nothing. My mother was too frightened to do so, for fear of reprisal. My mother suffered numerous injuries during our childhood—a broken nose, broken fingers, as well as other injuries such as bruised legs, bruised arms, etc.. Dad would deny that he had done anything the next morning.

When I was successful in calming him, he would go into the lounge room to eat his dinner. I can recall how revolting it was to watch him eat. He would either drop food on his clothes, or dribble down the side of his mouth. I used to cringe as I had to sit with him, feeling revolted by the whole picture. I used to think he was a dirty pig. When he had finished, Dad would call me to sit with him while he watched TV. I can recall feeling forced to sit with him in the lounge, with his arm around me, until he fell asleep. I would then very gently remove his arm and leave.

Dad would sometimes not return home before we went to bed. I used to lie awake on these nights waiting until he came home. I suffered from shocking nightmares. I vividly recall that the nightmares were of a man either standing beside my bed, or his face was right in my face. I would wake up screaming.

The eating disorder

I would say that I have suffered from a type of eating disorder since approximately the age of 16. I recall times of incredible anxiety, coupled with loss of appetite. This loss of appetite did not overly concern me because it seemed to be a good way of managing the anxiety problem. Later I married and had 2 children. When I became pregnant I was always hungry and saw that I had a good excuse to eat. I gained about 3.5 stone each time. This caused me a lot of anxiety and I again stopped eating and lost weight. Around this time my husband became involved with another woman. I can remember feeling the death of our relationship when I found them together. For me, marriage was for life. This exacerbated my eating problem more than any other time in my life. I exercised, took slimming tablets, laxatives, and ate.

It was shortly after this that my husband and his friend raped me one night after they had been out together drinking. I awoke to find them standing by the bed. I thought I was having another one of my nightmares and I became terrified. I was unable to say anything to them and eventually started crying. My husband later told me that if I did not wish them to have intercourse, I should have said something. I felt enormous guilt at this time because I wished I could have said something.

How have these events affected the quality of life for me in adulthood?

I found incredible difficulty in knowing how to relate to men without giving them the wrong signals. I always tried to be friendly to avoid any potentially aggressive situations. However, on reflection, this friendliness that I used to protect myself often became a cause for unwanted advances and which I felt I had no skills to handle. I used to feel so upset because I knew I should be able to deal with the situations as an adult, and yet I felt like a child in a woman's body, unable to speak up.

Around this time I tried to commit suicide because I felt unable to deal with everyday life. My life had become unmanageable. I went through bouts of drinking too much, being very eating disordered, suffering from constant anxiety and eventually, when I could no longer manage my life or the eating disorder, I was admitted to hospital for six months for treatment.

The ongoing effects of living with a physically violent and abusive father are still evident today. I have had an acute recurrence of panic attacks and the eating disorder due to a very traumatic event in my life. I have become more aware than ever before just how much my life has been impacted by the things of the past and the way in which I have learned to control my environment with dysfunctional behaviours. I struggle every day with the eating disorder—I wake up thinking about being too fat and go to bed at night feeling too fat. I feel angry when I have to deal with food because it seems to have such a huge control over me. I sink into despondency . . .

5
Eating disorders, pregnancy, and postpartum

Pregnancy is a major challenge to a woman's body weight and body image. During pregnancy changes take place slowly at first and then quite quickly as pregnancy progresses. The first noticeable change is the increase in the size of the breasts. These are like the premenstrual changes in fullness and tenderness familiar to many women but during pregnancy the breasts continue to enlarge. Some women with small breasts may be delighted with these changes while women who worry about the large size of their breasts may find these changes uncomfortable and feel self-conscious about their body image.

From very early in pregnancy changes in the hormones, produced by the placenta, prepare for the needs of the developing foetus. In early pregnancy the mother easily supplies the oxygen and nutrients for her developing foetus and can continue moderate amounts of low intensity exercise. As the demands made by the foetus increase the mother slows down her activities and body functioning. At this stage of pregnancy most women exercise very lightly, if at all, feel relaxed and 'not like doing very much'. This allows energy to be stored in the form of fat in the breasts, hips, and thighs. This 'passivity' of pregnancy is essential for the growth and development of the baby but has a few disadvantages for mothers; two of these are constipation due to decreased motility of the gut and excess weight gain if she does not eat a sensible diet.

Weight gain during pregnancy

Weight gain during pregnancy is necessary. Until recently it was believed the baby would derive all the energy and nutrition it required

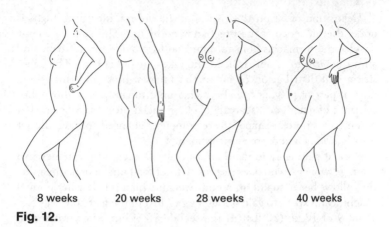

8 weeks   20 weeks   28 weeks   40 weeks

Fig. 12.

from its mother, even if the mother was in a state of starvation. There is now evidence to show that women who maintain low body weights and women who restrict their weight gain during pregnancy are more likely to give birth to a growth-retarded baby.

Doctors and midwives no longer recommend an ideal amount of weight to be gained during pregnancy, as this can be misleading and dangerous to the health and development of the baby, and the physical and psychological well-being of the mother. To understand weight gain during pregnancy it can be helpful to examine what contributes to the weight gain. The increased size of the breasts, the foetus and amniotic fluid that protects the foetus, the placenta that transports the oxygen and nutrients from mother to foetus and takes away the waste products, and the deposition of fat on the breasts, thighs, and hips are obvious contributors to most women. Less obvious is the 6–8 litres of fluid that are added to the body of the mother. Water is retained due to the action of the pregnancy hormones on the tissues of the body. Additional fluid is needed to make up the large increase in blood volume that is necessary to carry the oxygen and nutrients to the growing foetus. The approximate contributions of these factors to the overall weight gain of a woman of average weight and average height during pregnancy are given in Table 14. The actual amounts are very variable as every woman is different, and every baby is different.

Deposition of fat on the tissues of the breasts, hips, and thighs is under the influence of the pregnancy hormones. This store of energy ensures the woman is able to continue to provide for her baby and after the birth to be able to feed and take care of her baby. The deposition and distribution of fat to the breasts, hips, and thighs is a normal part of pregnancy. The media unfortunately only show photographs of glamorous, scantily clad, or naked pregnant women that obscure this normal shape or are computer changed to have the fat distribution of a non-pregnant woman.

Weight gain is more rapid after about 20 weeks of pregnancy. An 'average' woman, who does not restrict her food intake or act in a way that allows her to maintain a body weight which is below her normal weight, can expect to gain about 3 kg (7 lbs) in the first 20 weeks and about 9 or 10 kg (20 lbs) in the second 20 weeks. Many women, if they are weighed during pregnancy, will find their weight varies very widely and they do not follow the pattern suggested above. Most women gain 10–15 kg, average 12.5 kg (22–33 lbs average 27 lbs) during pregnancy.

The amount of weight a mother needs to gain in pregnancy will vary. Underweight women need to gain an amount of weight to give them a body weight before pregnancy in the normal weight range (BMI 19–25) and in addition the normal healthy weight gain expected during pregnancy. If the underweight mother tries to restrict her weight gain, particularly in early pregnancy, she may be failing to provide her infant with his or her optimal growth and development in her uterus. Overweight and obese women do not need to put on as

Table 14. Factors contributing to weight gain during pregnancy

The reasons for weight gain in pregnancy	Approximate percentage contribution to weight gain during pregnancy
Foetus and placenta	32%
Breasts and uterus	10%
Increase in blood volume	10%
Fat deposited	22%
Water retained	26%

much weight during pregnancy, probably as they already have reserves of energy to ensure development of their future infant. There is preliminary research to suggest that obese women, who do not suffer from any medical complications during pregnancy, do have small babies and that these babies may also not have reached their full growth potential.

Eating during pregnancy

The increased energy needs in pregnancy are modest. Most women will find they are eating slightly more, perhaps an extra glass of milk and an extra 2 slices of bread each day. The idea of 'eating for two' is incorrect and will lead to increases in fat being stored in the body in excess of the amount required for a healthy pregnancy. A woman who 'eats for two' will not be able to lose this excess weight and return to her prepregnancy weight in the year after her baby is born. Many women report that their eating and nutrition improves during pregnancy, they eat more regularly and eat more nutritious foods that they understand will help their baby thrive. About 20 per cent of women feel their eating deteriorates; usually in response to concerns about the amount of weight they are gaining. This may occur when women are weighed during their antenatal visits and then told how much weight they have gained. Other women may commence binge-eating when they try to adhere to the advice of some doctors who mistakenly believe weight gain during pregnancy should be 'as little as possible'.

Binge-eating and food cravings

Binge-eating can occur during pregnancy and for 7 per cent of women who have never suffered from an eating disorder this may be the first time they have experienced disordered eating. Binge-eating is more common in the second half of pregnancy. This is the time when the foetus is growing rapidly and making increasing demands on their mother for food. Women who have ignored the messages to eat more to supply the demands of their baby, either because they were occupied with other aspects of their busy life or were trying to prevent gaining 'too much weight' are likely to eat quickly and continue to eat once they start eating. This resembles binge-eating. Eating in response to this inadequate maternal food intake may explain some of the binge-eating of pregnancy. Binge-eating may also follow the nausea and vomiting of early pregnancy if, because of vomiting, insufficient energy was available for storage in the mother's body. Binge-eating may occur in subsequent pregnancies.

Other triggers to binge-eating may be boredom associated with decreased activity, worry about the future, and being preoccupied with thoughts of food. Craving for certain foods is common during pregnancy. These cravings are very diverse and vary from woman to woman. The foods may have a high water content such as watermelon or oranges, or be high in fat and carbohydrate such as pizza and Mexican food, or high in carbohydrate such as bananas. The foods craved may taste spicy, bland, bitter, or salty. It is thought that these cravings reflect the needs of the woman's body and eating these foods, in moderation, will provide her with the nutrients she is lacking.

Menstruation and contraception

Lack of menstrual periods (amenorrhoea) is not a safe method of contraception nor is being at low body weight or obese. Fertility is greatly reduced but even without menstrual periods women can ovulate and pregnancy can and does occur. If women suffering eating disorders are sexually active and if they do not desire pregnancy they need contraception. The menstrual cycle and menstruation are described on page 154.

Women with anorexia nervosa or bulimia nervosa may have been prescribed oral contraceptives for contraception or for hormone replacement to prevent loss of bone density (see Chapter 9). Women taking 'the pill', unless they are very emaciated, will experience bleeding via the vagina each month. This is called a 'withdrawal bleed'. When 'the pill' is taken as prescribed the 'pill' hormones are usually provided for 21 days and placebo (fake) tablets for 7 days of the 28-day pill pack. The menstrual-like bleeding occurs because the 'pill' hormones are stopped or 'withdrawn'. The occurrence of a 'withdrawal bleed does not mean menstruation and a normal ovulatory menstrual cycle will occur when 'the pill' is ceased. Women who commence oral contraception when they are having regular menses and then develop an eating disorder may find they are amenorrhoeic (no periods for 3 months or more) when they stop the 'pill'. If women recover from their eating disorder before stopping oral contraception menstruation is likely to occur.

Getting pregnant

Both underweight and overweight women and women with eating and exercise disorders may have difficulties falling pregnant. Women who desire fertility should be encouraged to accept help with their disordered eating before becoming pregnant. It may not be possible to achieve a 'cure' for the eating disorder before they wish to conceive but small changes in behaviour can help conception. When underweight women begin to increase their body weight and obese women lose some weight the levels of hormones involved in reproduction improve and ovulation can occur. Decreasing the frequency or ceasing methods of weight loss that are stressful to the body also improves the chances of pregnancy. Learning to eat regularly throughout the day and exercising sensibly may be sufficient for normal weight women, who are recovering from their eating disorder, to conceive.

Treatment of disordered eating can prevent the need for assisted conception. However if an eating disorder sufferer, in conjunction with her partner, feels recovery from her eating disorder will take too long or not be successful they can be reassured that assisted conception, although expensive and uncomfortable, is usually successful. Treatment with hormones used to induce ovulation, IVF (in vitro fertilisation), or one of the newer technologies will usually result in a pregnancy. Unfortunately these methods of assisted conception are more likely to result in miscarriage and several attempts may be needed. There are also risks with the treatment. Drugs used to induce ovulation may cause excessive ovarian enlargement (the ovarian hypersensitivity syndrome) which in some cases leads to abdominal pain, fluid in the abdomen, a fall in blood pressure, and in a few cases life-threatening blood coagulation changes. These changes are reversible for the majority of women.

Eating disorders and management during pregnancy

Women suffering from disordered eating are more likely to experience complications during their pregnancy. These difficulties include an increased risk of miscarriage, vomiting that requires treatment in hospital (hyperemesis gravidarum), gestational diabetes, pregnancy induced hypertension, and delivery of a small growth-retarded, premature, or large baby. After the birth postpartum haemorrhage, postnatal depression, and feelings of distress are common.

There is accumulating evidence being published in scientific journals to suggest that the uterine environment in which babies develop and grow may affect their quality of life as an adult. This warm, protective, and nurturing environment is influenced by maternal behaviours including her eating, drinking, and exercise. The uterine environment associated with the birth of a large for gestational age (LGA) infant may predispose this infant, if she is female, to breast cancer as an adult. Intrauterine growth-retarded infants born to mothers of low body weight are at increased risk of cognitive disorders and low birth weight babies may have a greater frequency of adult cardiovascular disease.

To ensure women with eating disorders give their babies the best possible start in life dietetic, psychological, and medical support must be available during their pregnancies. Each woman should be assessed by members of a multidiscipline team early in pregnancy, and introduced to people who can help her if she needs information or finds that her eating becomes a problem later in pregnancy. Most treatment will consist of reassurance, particularly about weight and shape issues and pregnancy symptoms, and support both during and after the birth. To help women suffering from eating disorders some suggestions have been made for health professionals to improve the quality of antenatal and postnatal care; these are shown in Table 15. The woman's partner or family should be included in the assessment and they should also be offered support during pregnancy and after childbirth.

A few women may need to stay in hospital to establish eating patterns that are compatible with adequate nutrition for both mother and her baby, or to correct electrolyte and fluid imbalances in the body that may arise from vomiting in early pregnancy and to treat obesity related medical problems.

Table 15. Suggestions for health professionals for the antenatal care of women with eating disorders

1. *Prepregnancy body weight.* Ask about the weight immediately before pregnancy and calculate the woman's BMI. If above 30 or below 18 the woman should be assessed very carefully and followed more intensely during pregnancy.

2. *Measure height.* The height given by women is not always accurate.

3. *Measure the body weight at some visits.* Explain to each woman you need to know her body weight during pregnancy, as this is one piece of information that tells you her baby is growing normally. Body weight is no longer measured routinely in many antenatal clinics, as women often do not like to be weighed.

4. *Ask women if they want to be told their body weight.* Ten to 20 per cent of pregnant women, particularly if they have an eating disorder, will become more preoccupied with thoughts of food and experience deterioration in their eating behaviour if they are told their weight. These women can be weighed with their back turned towards the scales. The person recording the weight must always be aware of the woman's wish to know or not to know.

5. *Assess nutrition, eating, and weight controlling behaviour.* A person who is experienced with nutrition during pregnancy and eating disorders should make this assessment. This assessment should be made as early in pregnancy as possible and again early in the third trimester. 'At risk' women should be followed throughout pregnancy and the first year after the birth.

6. *Assess exercise behaviour and lifestyle.* This assessment should examine the type and amount of exercise, including walking that may not be considered part of an exercise programme. The ability of the pregnant woman to change her behaviour and exercise lifestyle should be assessed, particularly in hot climates.

7. *Medications taken.* Most women try to avoid taking any medications when they are pregnant. Women with disordered eating patterns are more likely to smoke cigarettes for weight control and to take antidepressant medication. The progesterone only pill for contraception should be discussed with the woman.

8. *Nausea and vomiting.* Hyperemesis gravidarum is more common in women with eating disorders during pregnancy. Women with and without eating disorders admit to vomiting during pregnancy to feel better and prevent weight gain. Most women are able to decrease their frequency of vomiting when they know it may affect their baby.

Table 15. Suggestions for health professionals for the antenatal care of women with eating disorders (*continued*)

9. *Provide information about eating and body weight.* Information needs to be provided to women during and after each pregnancy. Most women are concerned about weight gain and weight loss; changes in body shape and the effect of changing their eating and exercise behaviour. This information needs to be readily available as the woman's experiences and concerns change during pregnancy, during breast-feeding, and during her adaptation to motherhood.

10. *Assess pre- and postnatal mood.* Women with a history of an eating disorder are more likely to experience mood disturbances and postnatal depression. The depressed mood may be present before and after pregnancy and sometimes not until 3 or 6 months after the birth.

11. *Breast-feeding.* Women may breast-feed because they believe this will aid weight loss after pregnancy. Women need to eat more while they are breast-feeding and adjust their eating patterns again after ceasing breast-feeding. The fatigue, lack of sexual interest, and lowering of mood associated with breast-feeding may modify the duration the woman chooses to breast-feed.

12. *Previous psychiatric history.* A previous history of psychological or psychiatric problems should be sought, particularly of depression, alcohol dependence, and eating disorders. Women with a previous history should be treated as 'at risk' during and for 12 months after pregnancy.

Anorexia nervosa and low prepregnancy body weight

Pregnancy, particularly if unexpected, may pose several challenges to women who are recovering or have recovered from anorexia nervosa. Some women look forward to the pregnancy, feeling that during pregnancy and when caring for a child they would be less preoccupied with body weight and eating and that 'pregnant women are allowed to be "fat"'. These women find being pregnant provides a relief from their eating and weight losing behaviours. Other women may become extremely distressed and anxious with the changes in their body image and report an exacerbation or no change in their eating disordered behaviours.

The desire to become pregnant can be sufficiently strong to induce some women to increase their weight and try to recover from anorexia nervosa or to increase their weight to achieve ovulation and pregnancy even if they return to low weight between each pregnancy. Other women prefer to have ovulation induced and accept assisted conception (see getting pregnant). During pregnancy anorexia nervosa sufferers may become distressed and feel they cannot put on weight, they may accept this and lose weight or allow themselves to gain a small amount of weight that they feel will be lost easily after the birth. Other women enjoy their pregnancy and gain the amount of weight necessary to ensure delivering a baby who has achieved its full growth potential before the birth.

Recently we studied healthy women who had delivered their first baby in the previous week. We found that 32 per cent of women who gave birth to a growth-retarded baby were suffering from an eating disorder, usually anorexia nervosa or an eating or exercise disorder involving low body weight. The mothers who were most 'at risk' of retarding the growth and development of their babies in the uterus were at a low BMI before pregnancy and failed to gain adequate weight during pregnancy although they felt that they were overeating during the pregnancy. Women who are at low body weight (BMI less than 19) at the time of conception and who fail to increase their body weight during pregnancy are more likely to give birth to a growth-retarded, low body weight baby. Babies who are of low body weight (LBW) when they are born may be growth retarded in utero or preterm. A growth-retarded baby is small for the number of weeks of pregnancy when it is born (or during pregnancy when it is measured during ultrasound examination) while a preterm baby is small because it is born too early (less than 37 weeks of pregnancy). Babies can be both growth retarded and preterm.

To avoid growth retardation of her baby a woman who is underweight should be helped to increase her body weight early in pregnancy. The woman may need help from a dietitian and reassurance from her physician to achieve an appropriate weight gain. This will include the weight she needed to gain before pregnancy to be at a prepregnancy weight in the normal body weight range (above BMI of 19) plus the normal healthy weight gain expected during a pregnancy.

Intrauterine growth retardation is also associated with smoking cigarettes. Many women smoke cigarettes to help control their body weight and maintain lower body weights (see page 17). In Australia approximately 11 per cent of pregnant women admit to smoking more than 15 cigarettes per day throughout pregnancy and 4 per cent continue to smoke during pregnancy to control their weight. Women who smoke and who are at low body weight need extra care during pregnancy, from both their physician and dietitian.

Bulimia nervosa

Unexpected and unwanted pregnancy is common and frequently followed by a planned abortion among women who have suffered from bulimia nervosa. If women make the decision to continue with

Case history: Anthea

Anthea had gained very little weight during her first pregnancy. In her second pregnancy she was repeating this pattern and sought help. After discharge from the Eating Disorders Unit, she wrote:

What a battle it's been trying to gain weight so that I can have a healthy baby and at the same time still have the desire to keep my weight down. As you know, I tried hard on my own but didn't have much success. After ten years of having an eating disorder, the fact that I was carrying a child was not strong enough for me to stop my behaviour. I kept thinking back to my first pregnancy—no morning sickness, healthy and fit the whole way through, and I gave birth to a perfectly healthy and beautiful baby girl—knowing that my weight gain and eating habits throughout that pregnancy were far from normal. But I was anxious the whole time that my lack of weight gain would harm the baby.

I knew that I couldn't take the same risks again and so spent eight weeks at the Unit. The time I spent there was more than helpful, although the separation from my baby and husband was more difficult than I had ever imagined.

My weight gain in hospital was quite considerable initially and quite difficult to come to terms with, so I had to keep remembering exactly why I was there. The sooner I came to terms with that, the sooner I'd be back at home with my family.

My first week home was quite difficult, the hardest thing being the rejection given me by my daughter. Daddy was her hero and I'd taken

Case history: Anthea (continued)

the back seat. Feeling very sorry for myself, I found myself quite depressed and very tempted to return to former eating habits. I must admit that I had some difficult moments but managed to fight these bad times.

After being home now for six weeks and with about ten weeks to go I feel so proud to be pregnant! I know that my weight gain has slowed down, but my eating habits are a lot more normal than in my first pregnancy which makes me very content and very ready for the birth of another baby.

The thing for me to remember is that after I've had this baby, my body isn't going to return to normal straight away. At this stage I don't know how I will react, but will face it when the time comes.

their pregnancy they can respond in various ways. Some may cease binge-eating and self-induced vomiting 'to protect their baby' or they may find these behaviours stop because they become relaxed about their body shape and weight and feel pregnancy provides 'an excuse not to look perfect'. Other women report that their eating disorder becomes worse, usually in the last third of pregnancy when they begin to worry about losing weight after the birth. If women are binge-eating and purging every day before pregnancy these behaviours can continue unchanged throughout the pregnancy and postnatal period.

Women who vomit a lot during the first 12 to 16 weeks of pregnancy or who induce vomiting during pregnancy, have a greater chance of delivering a lower birth weight baby. Their babies are less likely to be growth retarded when they are born but may be delivered earlier than expected, in other words they are born prematurely or are preterm. Bulimia nervosa sufferers are more likely to miscarry (spontaneously abort their foetus in the first half of pregnancy) and their baby may die just before or after the birth. Certainly women suffering from bulimia nervosa are more likely to experience an unwanted pregnancy and are more likely to seek to terminate their pregnancy than women who do not have an eating disorder.

Some bulimic women vomit more than their pregnancy would explain, they allow themselves to vomit in response to the nausea experienced by pregnant women 'to feel better', 'to get rid of the nausea', and to 'avoid weight gain'. A few women may need to be treated for their vomiting in hospital. This is called hyperemesis gravidarum. Whether women who have trained themselves to vomit easily after eating are more likely to have difficulties stopping themselves vomiting during pregnancy is unknown.

Obesity

Overweight and obese women do not all have eating disorders but a proportion binge-eat and may increase their weight excessively in pregnancy. Their patterns of binge-eating have been described in this chapter. Excess weight gain, greater than 16 kg during pregnancy, is difficult to lose in the year following the birth unless the woman is able to follow a strict menu plan and exercise. Natural weight loss after pregnancy is thought to be under genetic control so, if this is true, a few women who have gained less than 15 kg will also be unable to lose this weight without exercise and a reduced energy intake.

Women who are obese at the onset of pregnancy may require additional antenatal care, as they are more likely to develop complications during pregnancy including gestation diabetes mellitus and pregnancy induced hypertension. Pregnancy induced hypertension is diagnosed when a woman's blood pressure is increased above 140 systolic and 90 diastolic. Her blood pressure must be treated to prevent eclampsia developing (convulsions and coma). It may be necessary to deliver her baby early, by caesarean, if her blood pressure cannot be reduced. Modest weight loss by obese women in preparation for pregnancy can reduce the incidence of these complications.

Maternal obesity is associated with other difficulties in labour leading to caesarean section, postpartum haemorrhage, and poorer outcome of pregnancy. Morbidly obese women, and women who suffer from pregestational and gestation diabetes deliver large babies (LGA, large for gestational age). To reduce the risk of the birth of a LGA infant it is recommended that maternal weight gain during pregnancy should not exceed 12 kg or 25 lbs.

Obese women who deliver their first child are more likely to deliver a very preterm infant (less than 31 weeks of gestation) and have an increased risk of their foetus dying late in pregnancy. Poor weight gain during pregnancy may be associated with an increased risk of low birth weight and growth retarded babies to mothers who are obese. For this reason women who elect to have weight reduction operations are advised to use very safe methods of contraception during the rapid weight loss that follows the surgery. This is particularly important for those women who have failed to conceive because of their obesity, since fertility may increase following even a small loss of weight.

Past sufferers of eating disorders

During pregnancy women who have recovered from their eating disorder are similar to women who have never had disordered eating. They are not more likely to miscarry, lose their babies later in pregnancy, experience complications during pregnancy and the postnatal period, or to deliver large, preterm, or small babies.

Women with a past history of an eating disorder may find that during pregnancy they experience some of the previous disordered thoughts, fears, and preoccupation with food and body weight. This may account for the tendency of many 'recovered' anorexic and bulimic patients to gain less weight than expected during pregnancy.

It is not possible to predict if a woman who is recovering from disordered eating and exercise will be free from her problem during pregnancy. She may experience an improvement, an exacerbation, and a relapse, or report no change to her eating or exercise. One woman can respond in a different way during and after each of her pregnancies.

Postnatal distress and postnatal depression

Women suffering with anorexia nervosa and bulimia nervosa are more likely to seek help for distress and depression in the year after the birth of a child, particularly if it is their first child. In a recent study we found that women who are most at risk of postnatal mood problems are more likely to use dangerous methods of weight control such as self-induced vomiting or to binge-eat.

Women give a range of explanations for their postnatal problems. Unrealistic and idealised expectations of motherhood are common. They may have mistakenly believed that having a child would solve their problems by 'giving them something to think about apart from themselves', 'making their partner more loving', or 'having someone to love'. Many women do not realise what hard work it is to take care of a baby. Women who are depressed during pregnancy can remain depressed after pregnancy, and women with a previous history of depression are more likely to become depressed in the few years after the birth of a child. Postpartum depression is thought to result from the changes in hormones in a woman's body after giving birth, that affect the neurotransmitter chemicals in the brain that influence mood.

Women suffering from eating disorders need additional support during the postnatal period. Time away from her infant, reassurance she is coping well, practical information, and help coping with her child will decrease her distress. Mild exercise can help prevent depressed moods following childbirth, but for some women it may be suggested that they take antidepressant medication.

Breast-feeding

In Australia, and probably in other developed countries, infant-feeding practises for women with eating disorders have changed. Previously women with eating disorders were less likely to breast-feed, as they believed it would change their body shape and they would develop saggy breasts. This has changed and currently women believe they will lose body weight more quickly if they breast-feed, so most woman, who are conscious of their body weight and shape, breast-feed. It is true that a woman requires more energy (in the form of food) than her body needed during pregnancy if she is to breast-feed her baby. For her body to obtain this energy, she receives messages from the brain that tell her to eat more food and drink more fluid. Most women will find it extremely difficult to restrict their food intake at this time as they will experience constant thoughts about food and feel the need to eat and drink if they do try to limit their intake.

Some women find difficulty decreasing the amount of food eaten in the few weeks after lactation has stopped, for some women it may cause them to binge-eat or attempt starvation.

If women are not coping well because of fatigue and feeling down in mood and not enjoying breast-feeding they can be reassured and given permission to cease breast-feeding, particularly if women have breast-fed for 3 months or more. In a study of women without eating disorders we found that; immediately after ceasing breast-feeding even after 18 months of infrequent on-demand feeding women feel their mood improves, that they are less fatigued and more interested in sexual matters. Women may also associate the progesterone only 'pill' taken for contraception between pregnancies with a depressed mood.

Parenthood

Women's concerns about their eating behaviour and attitudes to body weight may interfere with their care of the child. The woman may be overly concerned about her child's weight and shape and this may transfer and affect the child's eating behaviour. Women who are trying to teach their children 'good eating habits' and prevent them from becoming 'overweight' may restrict the type and amount of food they give their children, these children may be hungry and feel different from their friends and they may steal food from other children's lunch boxes. Other women fear that their judgement of normal eating may be inaccurate and become over concerned that they may deprive their children of food or may inadvertently overfeed their infant.

Children become aware of mothers who do not eat with the family, who only eat once or twice a day, or who graze throughout the day. Children learn by example. Patients have reported preschool children asking 'why Mummy goes to the bathroom after dinner' or why she 'only eats in the kitchen and not with us'. From time to time the woman may relapse and hoard food or limit the amount of food available to the family. This may help the woman feel better but it can be detrimental to the family. She may also suffer swings in mood or depressed moods.

One of our patients wrote:

It is all coming together, gradually. I just hope that I am not going to do too much damage to my kids whilst I 'grow up' and that I have enough time left to enjoy being me and that the fears and depression and isolation never overwhelm my mind again. On the basis of past experience I suppose that's a lot to ask—but who would have believed that I would have two kids of my own either!

I hope that everyone who is trapped in anorexia nervosa or any other 'lonely obsessive trap', and who realizes their misery and wants to escape, finds someone to trust and help them, as I did.

Women suffering from bulimia nervosa may neglect their children and have difficulty forming a good relationship with them.

For example, in order not to be disturbed during an eating binge, she may put her child in a separate room and close the door so that she can ignore its cries. In the longer term, women who have recovered from bulimia nervosa tend to be overly anxious about their child's weight and appearance, which may in turn affect the child's development.

Women who still have active bulimia nervosa when their child reaches school age may avoid taking him to school or attending child-parent activities, and then try to make up to the children in other ways.

Esther's story demonstrates this. She has permitted us to have access to her diary. She writes:

I'll do it in the morning, stomach too sore, I'm too lethargic and miserable after today's episode.

Panic—another birthday party invitation. Will the kids get to go to this one or can I avoid getting out of the car to pick them up. 'Mummy is always sick', they say.

Sean and Angeline asked if we could go to gym on Saturday or Sunday to visit our old friends. Promised, and lied as usual, as if!!

Didn't take Sean to soccer training, couldn't bring myself to go out of the house.

It's Thursday and wow, I haven't binged since Monday, keep it up.

Panic, the days are getting warmer, and soon I'll have to drop the 'hiding' clothes (to avoid my fatness and shape to be seen by others).

The kids' sports carnival tomorrow, don't know what to do, I have to go, but I'm terrified. I don't want anyone to see me, and the way people look at me!! I feel so scared and vulnerable when I look like this.

Three days and haven't binged or eaten anything bad, except I ate enough vegetable stir fry to feed an army.

Asked kids how they would feel if I couldn't make it to the sports carnival—very upset. I'll have to go, just grin and bear it. Took Sean to training tonight, actually got out of the car to pick him up. Angeline does gym but she meets me at the car just outside, can't wait to watch her again like I used to. So frustrated, what madness!

Sports carnival day has arrived, have to go, it's going to be so hot today and I'm wearing winter clothes. How am I going to face today. I have been eating good, not bingeing most of the week and I feel fatter than I did at the beginning of the week, why do I always go through this transition of looking worse before I look better; but I feel better.

I actually went to the sports carnival, and lived through it, ha!! Looking around I didn't really feel like I looked different to everyone else, except more shy than usual. I have been eating a good three meals a day, except maybe too many vegetables, but at least it's only vegetables.

Day number seven. I actually thought I had this good eating down to a T—but what happened today; well I couldn't pick the kids up from school, couldn't step out of the house. I are everything that contained fat. I made sure of that. Dad picked the kids up for me (the car was overheating) ha ha. I was too disgusted to go out, my stomach too stretched to breath properly, all I could do was lay down and panic, full of panic, my mind ached with panic, what have I done and I know Dad will be here soon and my sisters just happened to pop over—that's all I needed. I had to control the kids, which I feel I can never do properly, hold back the tears, and control the panic till they left. I have left it too long, how am I going to bring it all up now, well I tried anyway, tried being the operative word. I have become hopeless at this for some reason, even though the belts I use seem to reach half way down my throat, to the point that it bleeds and is sore for days.

I should be taking Sean to study group this afternoon but how can I drag myself out of the house—by this stage I'm in a hysterical cry, panic, frenzy; you see I'm not that successful at bringing it up. My sister's son goes to study group and she just happens to ring and ask if I would like her to pick Sean up and take him, great, he doesn't miss out. Homework, the kids, can't concentrate on anything but my disgusting, pitiful, poor excuse for a mother.

Try again tomorrow.

Who wants to wake up?

Well, it is inevitable, I had to wake up this morning, car isn't going that well so I ring my sister to take the kids to school. I would have loved to go with them today to buy them some books which are on sale this week at the school library, but instead I pack some money in their pockets and off they go, mummy's car isn't working well you see—ha! Another excuse, I'm full of them.

The majority of women with a history of disordered eating respond well to their role as a mother and find it is a very positive experience.

6
Investigation of eating disorders

I don't want to be like this, but what I eat still rules my life so that at times every waking minute seems occupied with thoughts of food and the day passes in the measured times between when I last ate and when I'll eat again. I'm still plagued with guilt about everything I consume unless I nearly fast. I dream of the perfect day when I have no appetite, no thought, desire, or temptation for food or to eat. I often despair of ever finding a solution.

Weight loss and excessive weight gain may be caused by several physical and psychiatric conditions. For example, starvation causes emaciation, as does advanced terminal cancer and tuberculosis; gross obesity may be due to a brain tumour or to an endocrine disorder. Among psychiatric disorders, depression poses a diagnostic problem. Many women who have an eating disorder, particularly bulimia, show clinical signs of depression. However, when the woman first presents asking for help it may be unclear to the doctor or psychologist if the depression led to the eating disorder or if the eating disorder led to the depression.

It is important to exclude medical and psychiatric disorders when making a diagnosis of an eating disorder. This can be done by obtaining a good history and after an appropriate physical examination by a doctor. This examination includes careful measurements of the person's weight and height, so that the Body Mass Index can be calculated. An efficient, self report, computer-generated and computer-reported examination of eating and exercise behaviour attitudes and feelings has now been developed. This can provide the clinician with a printed report of the BMI, diagnoses, behaviour, attitudes, and feelings of the woman to refer to during the interview. This approach is helpful to women who have difficulty talking about themselves and women who can be more truthful when they provide embarrassing information about themselves to a computer rather than to their clinician.

Most people with eating disorders either have a fear of becoming fat, or are obese and perceive themselves as ugly, massive, undesirable, or flabby. Both groups have poor self-esteem and a poor body image. For this reason it is important for the health professional (who may be a doctor or a psychologist) to make a psychological evaluation of the woman before starting any treatment. There are several psychological tests, and the information obtained from these can be converted into mathematical scales to help in this evaluation, each test having its adherents. Many of the tests are complex and the findings contradictory. Before deciding if any psychological tests are to be made, it may help to ask a few simple questions. But before they are asked, the appearance of the woman seeking help may determine which questions should be asked. As well as estimating her body size, other observations may be made. Is she wearing clothes which reveal her body shape or has she chosen loose-fitting garments to try to hide her body shape and weight? Does she have calluses on the back of her fingers? These may be associated with self-induced vomiting. Are her fingers and feet puffy? These signs may occur following the consumption of large amounts of food over a short period of time. Are her teeth discoloured or damaged? These conditions may follow frequent episodes of self-induced vomiting.

The purpose of the questions is to try to establish whether the patient is prepared to alter her eating behaviour, to lose or gain weight, and if she has sufficiently high motivation and fortitude to make the changes. If her motivation is low, a great deal of time will be expended, both by the health professional and the patient, with little benefit.

The following twenty questions have been tested and found to be helpful for health professionals in establishing someone's motivation to change her disordered eating behaviour. (As the questions are used by health professionals we use the term 'patient' in the rest of this chapter.)

We believe that the questions are also helpful for a reader who has an eating disorder to look more deeply into her attitudes and beliefs about her eating behaviours. You may find it helpful to write down your answer to each question and read it again a week or two later.

1. Do you really want to change your eating behaviour?

Even if a patient is unwilling to make changes in her eating behaviour at the time she seeks help, it is important that the health professional offers her support and provides a contact for her in the future. Some women take up to three years before they are ready to accept help for their eating disorder. There are a number of reasons for this. In mild cases the woman's acceptance of her present behaviour may outweigh the long-term consequences of emaciation or obesity. This implies that in some cases the person has to get worse, becoming even more emaciated, or more obese, or more disordered in her eating, before she is sufficiently motivated to accept treatment. In extreme cases when the illness may threaten her life, pressure must be placed on her to accept treatment.

Some women deny that their problem is one of disordered eating behaviour. These women insist that they can gain or lose weight easily if they want to, and after admitting that they binge-eat or induce vomiting, say that they could easily stop the bahaviour if they wanted to. In other words they, too, are ambivalent about starting treatment. One strategy to suggest to these women is that if they wish they can try to change their eating behaviour on their own, but to recommend that they should return four weeks for evaluation. The first page of the Eating and Exercise Examination by computer (EEE-C) is shown for four women on pages 96–99. During this period nearly regularly for all the women will have continuing failed to change their disordered eating and may be more ready to accept treatment.

2. What is your occupation?

Certain jobs which involve business entertaining, catering, extensive travelling, shift work, or long periods of relative inactivity and boredom, may frustrate the woman's attempts to change her eating behaviour. Knowledge of the patient's occupation helps the health professional to suggest strategies for resisting the compulsion to eat or to diet. Occupations which require the patient to be thin, such as fashion modelling or ballet dancing, have to be accepted, and treatment may have to be modified so that the desired weight fits in with the occupation. Another example is the woman whose occupation is involved with food preparation or who is a waitress, because her occupation may reinforce her preoccupation with food.

3. What is your weight now?

Assessment of the patient's current weight enables the health professional to estimate how long it will take for the woman to achieve a realistic weight if her motivation is high and if she adheres to the recommended menu plan, whether this is to achieve refeeding or weight reduction. Knowledge of the woman's present weight may also give some indication about further medical investigations which should be made to avoid aggravating a possible vitamin deficiency or a metabolic disturbance, such as low blood potassium, which could cause cardiac arrest.

4. What weight would you like to achieve?

It is important for this to be discussed as the patient may have unrealistic expectations, which may frustrate her attempts to change her eating behaviour and may require modification. It is also helpful to explore the reason a particular weight was selected as the 'desirable' personal weight, if she is to recover from her eating disorder.

A woman may select a body weight which is below the range at which she can be sure to have recovered from her eating disorder. In other words she persists with her disordered eating to remain at her chosen weight. Other women, particularly if they are obese, may choose a body weight which is inappropriately low for her, simply because she has been told that weight is 'ideal' for her by a friend or the weight-loss industry.

The answer to this question also enables a treatment plan to be developed by the woman and her health professional. For example, if an obese woman has tried and learnt that starvation or yo-yo dieting is no good for her, the treatment plan has to address these issues.

5. What is the heaviest you have ever been?

This question establishes whether the person has previously attempted to reduce, or to increase, her weight; whether she failed or achieved partial success; and how she coped.

6. What is the lowest weight you reached?

The question has greater applicability to people who have anorexia nervosa and gives an indication of weight changes, at least those reported by the patient.

7. Have you maintained your weight over a period of at least six months without much effort?

This question gives a reasonable indication of a weight range which the patient could aim for, and it may help her recognize that she can maintain a body weight without being preoccupied with food.

As many women believe that their weight should be the 'ideal weight' proclaimed in many articles in women's magazines, it may be helpful to her to introduce the concept of a desirable weight-range as defined by the BMI, and dissuade her from seeking an ideal weight.

8. How do you think changing your weight will change your lifestyle?

Many patients try to generalize in answer to this question saying that 'I'll probably feel better' or 'I read that I should lose weight'. The question requires to be answered more specifically, and the patient should try to state clearly what things she hopes to do after weight change which cannot be done while she is emaciated or obese. It may help the patient if she makes a list of the reasons why she wants to gain or to lose weight. She may find difficulty in answering this question at the beginning of treatment, but later, with more insight into her eating disorder, this may help her to understand her eating problem. As an example, a patient who has anorexia nervosa who changes her weight may feel that she will lose control, not only of her eating behaviour but of her life-style, and may also lose the feeling of 'safety' she had when her body weight was low.

9. Are you trying to lose weight at present?

If the answer is yes, it is important to establish exactly what the diet contains, and how rigorous the patient has been in keeping to it. For example, many obese people try new fashionable 'fad' diets but the diet is not really effective and the dieter has insufficient motivation to keep to it. Information about the patient's chosen diet is even more valuable when she has anorexia nervosa or bulimia. Starvation diets are more likely to end in an episode of binge-eating than 'sensible' diets, rather in the way a person who misses breakfast and lunch because of work or other circumstances feels hungry when dinner-time approaches and is likely to eat more at dinner than normal. It is

EEE-C Clinical Report

(only to be used as an adjunct to clinician's assessment) © *Suzanne Abraham*

CODE: RIA184	DATE: 12/06/98	NAME: Gwyneth

BACKGROUND INFORMATION

Birthdate	26/02/82
Sex	F
Age	16
Marital Status	Single
Number of Children	0
Current height (m)	1.67
Current weight (kg)	41.45
BMI	14.9
Lowest ever BMI	14.7
Age at Lowest BMI	16
Highest ever BMI	20.1
Age at Highest BMI	14
Menstrual Status	Secondary Amenorrhoea
Meal Status	3
Physical Activity	Non specific

Current Medical Conditions	Nil
Current Medication	Zoloft
Current Psychiatric Conditions	Obssessive Compulsive Disorder

EXAMINATION SCORES (range 0-20)

Undereating Behaviour	13
Eating Behaviour for Weight or Shape	12
Overeating Behaviour	5
Eating Attitudes	14
Exercise Attitudes	17
Weight Feelings	15
Shape Feelings	17
Psychological Feelings	9
Total Average EEE Score	13
Body Appearance Rating (range 0-10)	3
Desired BMI	16.1

BEHAVIOURAL CRITERIA FULFILLED

Objective Binge	NO
Subjective Binge	YES
Objective Binge Eating	NO
Subjective Binge Eating	NO
Purging	YES
Non-Purging for Bulimia Nervosa	N/A
Excessive Exercise	NO
Excessive Exercising	NO

DIAGNOSTIC CRITERIA FULFILLED *

in the previous three months and previous month	3 months	1 month
Anorexia Nervosa	YES	YES
Anorexia Nervosa - not for Weight or Shape	N/A	N/A
Bulimia Nervosa	N/A	N/A
Exercise Disorder	NO	NO
Eating Disorder - Binge Eating Disorder	N/A	N/A
Eating Disorder - not otherwise specified	N/A	N/A

* Postpubertal

EEE-C Clinical Report

(only to be used as an adjunct to clinician's assessment)   © *Suzanne Abraham*

Printed on 27/11/98 14:00:13
Page 1
EEE-C v4.0

CODE: T0105	DATE: 31/03/98	NAME: Mary

BACKGROUND INFORMATION

Birthdate	14/10/65
Sex	F
Age	33
Marital Status	Married
Number of Children	0
Current height (m)	1.54
Current weight (kg)	44
BMI	18.6
Lowest ever BMI	16
Age at Lowest BMI	20
Highest ever BMI	23.2
Age at Highest BMI	24
Menstrual Status	Regular
Meal Status	3
Physical Activity	Athletic training program

Current Medical Conditions	Nil
Current Medication	Nil
Current Psychiatric Conditions	Nil

EXAMINATION SCORES (range 0-20)

Undereating Behaviour	9
Eating Behaviour for Weight or Shape	9
Overeating Behaviour	0
Eating Attitudes	5
Exercise Attitudes	19
Weight Feelings	7
Shape Feelings	10
Psychological Feelings	7
Total Average EEE Score	8
Body Appearance Rating (range 0-10)	7
Desired BMI	17.7

BEHAVIOURAL CRITERIA FULFILLED

Objective Binge	NO
Subjective Binge	NO
Objective Binge Eating	NO
Subjective Binge Eating	NO
Purging	NO
Non-Purging for Bulimia Nervosa	N/A
Excessive Exercise	YES
Excessive Exercising	YES

DIAGNOSTIC CRITERIA FULFILLED *

in the previous three months and previous month	3 months	1 month
Anorexia Nervosa	NO	NO
Anorexia Nervosa - not for Weight or Shape	NO	NO
Bulimia Nervosa	NO	NO
Exercise Disorder	YES	YES
Eating Disorder - Binge Eating Disorder	NO	NO
Eating Disorder - not otherwise specified	NO	YES

* Postpubertal

EEE-C Clinical Report

(only to be used as an adjunct to clinician's assessment) © Suzanne Abraham

CODE: A00100	DATE: 13/08/98	NAME: Sally

BACKGROUND INFORMATION

Birthdate	20/07/73
Sex	F
Age	25
Marital Status	Single
Number of Children	0
Current height (m)	1.6
Current weight (kg)	46
BMI	18.0
Lowest ever BMI	15.6
Age at Lowest BMI	24
Highest ever BMI	21.9
Age at Highest BMI	14
Menstrual Status	Oral contraception
Meal Status	3
Physical Activity	Non specific

Current Medical Conditions	Nil
Current Medication	prosac
Current Psychiatric Conditions	Nil

EXAMINATION SCORES (range 0-20)

Undereating Behaviour	8
Eating Behaviour for Weight or Shape	7
Overeating Behaviour	14
Eating Attitudes	18
Exercise Attitudes	9
Weight Feelings	17
Shape Feelings	19
Psychological Feelings	18
Total Average EEE Score	15
Body Appearance Rating (range 0-10)	3
Desired BMI	16.4

BEHAVIOURAL CRITERIA FULFILLED

Objective Binge	YES
Subjective Binge	NO
Objective Binge Eating	YES
Subjective Binge Eating	NO
Purging	YES
Non-Purging for Bulimia Nervosa	N/A
Excessive Exercise	NO
Excessive Exercising	NO

DIAGNOSTIC CRITERIA FULFILLED *

in the previous three months and previous month	3 months	1 month
Anorexia Nervosa	NO	NO
Anorexia Nervosa - not for Weight or Shape	NO	NO
Bulimia Nervosa	YES	YES
Exercise Disorder	NO	NO
Eating Disorder - Binge Eating Disorder	N/A	N/A
Eating Disorder - not otherwise specified	N/A	N/A

* Postpubertal

EEE-C Clinical Report

(only to be used as an adjunct to clinician's assessment) © *Suzanne Abraham*

Printed on 18/02/99 10:18:28
Page 1
EEE-C v4.0

CODE: OC013	DATE: 13/10/98	NAME: Katie

BACKGROUND INFORMATION

Birthdate	29/01/71
Sex	F
Age	28
Marital Status	Single
Number of Children	0
Current height (m)	1.7
Current weight (kg)	140
BMI	48.4
Lowest ever BMI	28.4
Age at Lowest BMI	16
Highest ever BMI	48.4
Age at Highest BMI	27
Menstrual Status	Regular
Meal Status	3
Physical Activity	Limited for medical reasons

Current Medical Conditions	asthma
Current Medication	prednisone, zoloft, pulmicort, ventolin, flicitase, tazac, beconase, oxis
Current Psychiatric Conditions	Nil

EXAMINATION SCORES (range 0-20)

Undereating Behaviour	5
Eating Behaviour for Weight or Shape	4
Overeating Behaviour	17
Eating Attitudes	14
Exercise Attitudes	6
Weight Feelings	17
Shape Feelings	20
Psychological Feelings	19
Total Average EEE Score	14
Body Appearance Rating (range 0-10)	0
Desired BMI	28.4

BEHAVIOURAL CRITERIA FULFILLED

Objective Binge	YES
Subjective Binge	NO
Objective Binge Eating	YES
Subjective Binge Eating	NO
Purging	NO
Non-Purging for Bulimia Nervosa	N/A
Excessive Exercise	NO
Excessive Exercising	NO

DIAGNOSTIC CRITERIA FULFILLED *

in the previous three months and previous month	3 months	1 month
Anorexia Nervosa	NO	NO
Anorexia Nervosa - not for Weight or Shape	NO	NO
Bulimia Nervosa	NO	NO
Exercise Disorder	NO	NO
Eating Disorder - Binge Eating Disorder	YES	YES
Eating Disorder - not otherwise specified	N/A	N/A

* Postpubertal

also useful to find what the diet contains, as some 'health' foods contain considerable amounts of sugar, and many obese people do not consider beverages as food, although they contain sugar. Even 'low-energy' foods and drinks provide a considerable amount of energy if the person eats or drinks quantities of them, believing that they will not put on weight.

Many women with eating disorders lose their perception of how much they need to eat, or not to eat, if they wish to maintain a constant weight. Obese people tend to over-estimate their food needs, while patients with anorexia nervosa tend to under-estimate how much they should eat to maintain a constant weight. Bulimia nervosa patients usually under-estimate their requirements because they do not include the food eaten during a binge as normal eating.

10. Have you previously tried dieting to lose or to gain weight?

If the person has dieted previously and has failed to gain or to lose weight while dieting or has kept to the diet for only a short time, it is important to establish this fact, as well as finding out why previous attempts at dieting were abandoned.

11. Have you used any other ways apart from dieting to lose weight?

People who have failed to lose weight because they have not kept to their menu plan often try other methods such as self-induced vomiting, or laxative or diuretic abuse, or excessive exercise in an attempt to lose weight. This applies to bulimia patients, anorexia nervosa patients, and obese patients. In fact over 40 weight-losing behaviours were reported in a study made in Sydney (Table 3, p. 13). Some of the methods are potentially dangerous, but most patients only resort to them when simpler methods have apparently failed. It may help the patient understand her eating disorder if the reason why the methods failed to work is talked about or thought about. As some people feel ashamed of using these methods it may be difficult for some patients to admit that they have used them. But the patient and her therapist should try to explore them, since much of the management of eating disorders is directed to changing eating and weight-losing behaviours. The question also enables the physician to decide if further medical and laboratory investigations are needed.

12. If you keep strictly to your menu plan, how quickly do you think that you will gain weight if you have a weight-losing eating disorder or will lose weight if you are obese?

A woman who is trying to gain weight will find it relatively easy to increase her body weight by eating a little more food in the first two weeks of her new menu plan, but it is unrealistic for her to expect that her weight gain will continue unless she progressively increases her food intake.

Similarly in the case of an obese woman, unrealistic expectations about losing weight (usually obtained from reading about 'fad' or crash diets) can be clarified by asking the question. For example, many obese people know that on a strict diet it is relatively easy to lose 3 kg (7 lbs) in the first week, but expect to be able to continue losing weight at this rate which is unrealistic (this is discussed further on p. 265). They find that they do not lose weight rapidly after the first week and may give up the diet assuming that it is 'no good'. It also helps the patient to know that the weekly weight loss or weight gain may fluctuate even though she has adhered to her menu plan. A person who says 'I have only to look at food to put on weight' is playing games with herself, and is either eating snacks or practising 'picking behaviour'; so is a person who says to herself that 'a piece of cake, or a chocolate, won't do any harm'—and goes on eating pieces of cake and chocolates.

13. An obese woman may be asked: 'Do you expect to lose weight without dieting?'

The question may seem stupid at first. Of course, the person will answer that she does not: but when the subject is explored further it will be found that most people seek magic cures for obesity or for losing weight while continuing to binge-eat. Many of these women spend considerable quantities of money following 'fad' diets or attending various courses guaranteeing painless weight reduction.

14. Are you taking any medication at present?

This question is designed to determine what medication the patient has been given, why the medications were prescribed or bought, and whether they are really needed. It explores the matters raised in question 11.

15. Tell me about your family?

The question is deliberately vague. It seeks to determine if the parents of the patient were fat; whether siblings or children are fat; what sort of life the family leads; what pressures are put on the person by the other family members; who does the cooking and who the shopping; if the family eat meals together; if other family members are dieting. Family dynamics may have a considerable influence on the patient's opinion of herself and disclosure may help in changing eating behaviour.

The question also may lead to a discussion about how the patient relates to her family and whether there is any conflict between members of the family. It is important young women with anorexia nervosa can relate to a supportive person, usually this is her mother but in some cases another family member or family friend may need to be contacted.

This question may help to clarify if the person has inherited 'fat genes' (see page 247), since if she has, it may be necessary to modify treatment goals.

16. Tell me about your lifestyle

The information obtained from this question enables the therapist to decide on the strategy which is most likely to succeed in inducing the woman to change her eating behaviour and to persist with the new eating habit. It will also help her to recognize there may be a need for her to change her lifestyle, including where and with whom she is living, if she is to recover.

17. How do you feel about yourself?

This question seeks to explore how the woman perceives herself in relation both to herself and to others. In other words it tries to find out about her self-esteem.

18. Have you ever had any unpleasant physical or sexual experience?

There is increasing evidence that a number of women who have an eating disorder may have been abused physically and sexually during childhood. This question gives the person the opportunity to talk about such an experience and to discuss any physical and mental abuse that may have occurred within the family.

19. Have you had any problems becoming pregnant?

Some women may be asked this question, as infertility is not uncommon amongst women with an eating disorder, and women being investigated for infertility are not usually asked about their eating behaviour. A woman who has an eating disorder or is recovering from an eating disorder and who becomes pregnant requires increased care in pregnancy and after childbirth (see Chapter 5).

20. Have any of your family been treated for any psychological or psychiatric problem?

There is increasing evidence that a proportion of young women with a weight-losing eating disorder have a parent or a close relative who has received help for a psychological or psychiatric problem, particularly depression, alcohol dependence, or an eating disorder. All the eating disorders described in this book occur more commonly in families, and are more common in identical twins when compared with fraternal twins. This suggests there are a range of genetic factors that play a role in the development of the eating disorders.

7 The general management of eating disorders

When this all started, I used to always use a knife to eat an apple, and a tea-spoon to eat cereal or dessert—I suppose it took longer, and therefore felt as if I was eating more. I always left a bit of potato / rice / noodles on my plate, no matter how much was served to me—as a test of willpower. The whole exercise of putting on weight, to me, is a breakdown of my iron willpower, because I know only too well that I enjoy eating. That is what still revolts me—the amount of food actually to be consumed in order to put on one stone. I've always maintained that I would so much prefer to have one stone in weight 'sewn' on instead of having to 'eat' it on.

Eating disorders occur because a person loves food and either seeks to control this love rigorously (anorexia nervosa) or intermittently (bulimia nervosa, binge-eating disorder, and eating disorders not otherwise specified) or has a lack of control over the amount of food eaten (obesity—although many other factors are involved in obesity, as we discuss on pages 246–51). It follows from this observation that the reversion of an eating disorder to 'normal' eating depends on several decisions. The first is that the person perceives that she has an eating disorder. The second is that the person believes that if the disordered eating continues it may cause a serious problem to her lifestyle or to her health, or both. In other words, she has to decide that the benefit, or reward, of changing the disordered eating behaviour exceeds that of the cost of continuing with it, at a physical, psychological, and social level. Having made these decisions, she has to experience or show a readiness to change her present eating habits. This implies that she will accept the help given, but understands that the change will only occur if she is prepared to achieve the change herself. It is relatively easy to lose (or to gain) weight so that it lies within the desirable range: it is much harder to *maintain* the weight within the desirable range.

Who should help a person who has an eating disorder?

Once someone has accepted that she or he has an eating disorder and has decided to seek help, the choice of the helper may be the person's family doctor, psychiatrist, a dietitian, an eating disorder specialist, or a multidisciplinary team, which includes a dietitian, a psychologist, and a medical specialist. If her health is so bad that admission to hospital is required, the most successful results occur if she is admitted to a specialized Eating Disorders Unit, in the case of anorexia nervosa and bulimia nervosa, or to an Obesity Unit in the case of severe obesity.

Self-help manuals

Well-motivated patients who are not severely emaciated or grossly obese can choose to use a self-help manual (see Further Reading) or may be managed by their family doctor and a dietitian, but if improvement is not obtained within a few weeks, referral to a specialist is recommended.

The patient's general health and physical condition is evaluated, and laboratory tests made. The opportunity is then taken to talk with the patient explaining possible approaches for treatment, and that the disorder, whether it is anorexia nervosa, bulimia nervosa, or obesity takes time to be 'cured'. Miracle cures do not work. This means that the patient and the therapist will be in contact for months or years.

Self-help groups

Many women who experience an episode of disordered eating can receive help in the community. The self-help groups which help women achieve a loss of weight (such as Weight Watchers International, TOPS—taking off pounds sensibly, Overeaters Anonymous) are firmly established. Self-help groups for women with anorexia nervosa and bulimia nervosa are increasing in number in many countries. Providing that these groups are properly organized and run by responsible people they provide great help to many women.

Self-help groups have many advantages: (1) the leaders of the group have been able to alter their own eating habits and have achieved and maintained their weight goal: they are therefore able to serve as a model for the other members of the group; (2) the person finds it easy to join and to leave the group (this may be more difficult in treatment by a therapist, as she may feel an obligation to the therapist); (3) the group exerts a 'dynamic effect' which may help the person counter the psychological and social pressures which encourage relapse; (4) the method helps the person feel that she has achieved the changes of eating behaviour by her own efforts without a 'professional' taking over her treatment, although this negative effect is reduced if the professional is well-trained, skilled, and empathetic; (5) the person is not converted into a 'patient' with a 'disease'; (6) usually the courses provided by self-help groups are cheaper than those provided by health professionals, a factor which may be of some importance for compliance; and (7) some groups, notably those which help women with anorexia nervosa and bulimia, have people who are accessible at all times to help a woman who perceives herself to be in 'crisis'.

Recently people involved in self-help groups have obtained better training and the groups are more effective in helping women with disordered eating. Self-help groups may not be appropriate to help women who have a severe eating disorder, or a complicating medical or psychiatric problem. However, most responsible self-help groups 'screen' women with an eating disorder and recommend that women whose eating disorder is severe or who have a psychological or a medical problem receive additional help from a medical specialist.

Self-help groups have some dangers. The members of the group may teach each other bad habits, such as self-induced vomiting, or to compete to be the worst or best in the group. They may reinforce the woman's preoccupation with weight and food. They may have no routine assessment procedures to determine if the person needs to seek the help of a specialist. They may indirectly persuade the woman to keep her eating disorder so that she can continue to obtain the support of the group for other problems which she may have.

Internet treatment

Some therapists are including email contact with their patients as an adjunct to therapy; this is of great assistance to people who live in isolated areas in countries such as Australia and Canada. Assessment of the eating disorders via the Internet is also available.

Women with eating disorders have mixed feelings about the helpfulness of the current, easily accessed, eating disorder websites. Reading other women's experiences can be helpful and supportive or they can be destructive and teach new 'tricks' to help people avoid eating and lose weight. Chat lines can produce competitiveness and sensationalism, with participants trying to be the 'best' at their eating disorder. In the quest of 'a cure' many of our patients report becoming obsessed and preoccupied with Internet searches and chat lines to the detriment of their study and sleep.

Trained health professionals are developing eating disorder programmes with supervised chat lines. These programmes are expected to become available for small groups of people who have been clinically assessed and considered suitable for this approach. These provide positive self-help as the therapist is aware of each person's progress, the chat lines are supervised, and the therapists know the history of each participant. It combines group therapy with self-help whilst maintaining the anonymity of the participants. The effectiveness of this approach has not yet been assessed.

Local chat lines for women seeking information about treatments for chronic obesity can be extremely helpful, particularly if people are contemplating surgery. Those who have experienced surgery can help by providing information about different surgeons; there appears to be general disapproval of the surgeons who offer one visit only before the surgery, no dietetic and psychological assessment before, and no medical, dietetic, and psychological follow-up. Chat lines can also provide information about personal experiences of different 'magical' weight-losing methods and prevent people spending money on useless 'cures'.

Day-patient treatment

Once she has absorbed the information, she has to make a decision with the advice of her doctor (who may have to over-rule her if she is very ill) whether it is best for her to be treated as an out-patient or as a 'day-patient'; or whether to be admitted to hospital, to an Eating Disorder Unit or to an Obesity Unit.

Out-patient treatment

Unless the person is very ill, out-patient (ambulant) treatment or day-patient treatment is preferable for nearly all obese patients, for most women who have bulimia nervosa, and for some women who have anorexia nervosa. During ambulant treatment the patient usually makes progress, but if she does not improve, in-patient hospital treatment becomes necessary.

These matters are discussed later in the chapters related to the particular eating disorder.

Managing eating disorders

The aims of the treatment of someone with an eating disorder are:

(1) to persuade her to achieve and accept a weight which lies in the normal range (BMI 19–24.9) or a higher realistic weight if she is obese;

(2) to help her to learn or relearn 'normal eating';

(3) to help her gain insight into her eating behaviour and why the behaviour is persisting;

(4) to educate her about nutrition and normal eating and dispel myths about food and eating;

(5) to persuade her to stop using behaviours which are potentially dangerous;

(6) to help her overcome any problems in her life which may be aggravating the eating behaviour or preventing her recovery;

(7) to help her alter, or modify her lifestyle, if appropriate.

Table 16. How women with an eating disorder describe 'normal' eating

- when in company, eating slowly and finishing last, seeing how long I can stretch out the meal;
- when alone, eating quickly so that I get rid of it and don't enjoy it;
- saying no to food;
- filling up on fluids before meals;
- cutting up and dissecting my food to show I am in control;
- sticking to rigid eating times—too bad if you miss it;
- only eating 'healthy' foods, i.e. diet and fat-free foods;
- disguising the flavour of tasty foods so that they taste nasty;
- going on an eating binge;
- making food the focus of my day.

If the individual is to achieve the needed change she requires motivation, fortitude, persistence, and a continuing stimulus to change. This will only be achieved when she becomes aware of the factors—physiological, psychological, social, and familial—which induce her to continue her disordered eating. She also needs to become aware that what triggered the disordered eating habit is not necessarily the reason why it is continuing. For example, if a disturbed family relationship was one of the factors which led to the onset of anorexia nervosa, it may be necessary not only to explore this relationship but also to use other treatments. She may have to learn that although she has an intense fear of becoming fat, it is safe for her to try to increase her weight, and that she will not lose control of her eating and other behaviour. On the other hand, unless a grossly obese individual can be induced to lose her urge to eat, starting a strict diet may lead her to take one of two actions. First, she may give in to her urge to eat and so break her diet. At first the food gives her pleasure, but then guilt may follow and lead to depression. Alternatively, she may keep to her diet and suffer 'stress' because she does not accede to her urge to eat. This can lead to anger, frustration, or depression. If an obese person continues eating because of loneliness, boredom, or stress at work this must be examined.

As far as is possible the patient and her therapist have to agree to try and be honest with each other. The problem is that patients with eating disorders tend to 'play games' and to manipulate the therapist. In spite of this the patient should try to answer honestly that she is complying with the menu plan they have jointly chosen and should try to discuss how her altered eating behaviour is affecting other behaviour. As it is important to 'track' changes in behaviour as well as of weight during treatment the patient must be able to have confidence in and trust the therapist.

Eating behaviour and a mood diary

It often helps the woman to keep a daily diary of her moods and eating behaviour. She fills in the diary every night before going to bed. A diary which we use for patients who have bulimia nervosa binge-eating disorder or who purge, starve, overexercise, or feel they binge eat is shown in Table 17 (page 111). The diary also permits the woman to see the associations between her feelings, moods, and eating behaviour, to observe changes in her eating behaviour, and to note changes with her menstrual cycle.

Often when a patient feels that she is not improving in spite of treatment, checking back in the diary and talking about it with her therapist shows that her feeling is false and that she is improving.

During the recovery period, some women who have bulimia nervosa may observe by referring to the diary that they change from recording binge-eating to recording overeating. In other words, the nature of the binge has changed and the decision to eat or not to eat has been recognized. Later when the woman finds that her weight is not increasing she will stop recording 'overeating'. For some women, knowing that they have to record their binge-eating or vomiting may be sufficient for them to change their behaviour.

Eating behaviour and the food diary

A food diary (Table 18) is often helpful in the early stages of treatment if the woman has bulimia nervosa or is obese. The diary is designed to help the woman reduce her preoccupation with body weight, body shape, and food. However it is not usually helpful if the woman has anorexia nervosa, as it may increase her preoccupation with food and hinder her recovery. The diary should not be kept for long periods of time as, paradoxically, it may increase the woman's preoccupation with food, which is contrary to the aims of treatment.

In the diary the woman records everything that she eats and drinks and her feeling about it, which gives her insight into her eating behaviour. The diary is also helpful to the dietitian, who can make suggestions to help the woman slowly acquire a normal eating behaviour.

We should add that some women will not be ready to complete the food diary as they do not wish to admit to the frequency and severity of their inappropriate eating behaviour at an early stage of treatment.

Changes in lifestyle

It is important for the patient continually to be aware that changes in lifestyle are as important as changes in weight and that the two are inter-linked. During treatment the woman needs to become aware that the decision to change her eating behaviour to achieve and to

Table 17. Eating behaviour and mood diary

ID:　　　　Date commenced:　　　　Date LMP:

day	1	2	3	4	5	6	7	8	9	10	11	12	13	14
Today I:					0 = no, 1 = yes, 2 = a lot									
ate appropriately														
tried to restrict food intake														
tried to avoid eating														
overexercised														
binge-ate														
overate														
starved														
induced vomiting														
Today I felt:					0 = not at all, 1 = a little, 2 = a lot									
good														
content (with self)														
sad/depressed														
confused														
loss of control														
tense/agitated														
like binge eating														
like vomiting														
no. std. glasses alcohol														
no. cigarettes smoked														
menses present														
OC taken*														

* OC oral contraceptive

Table 18. Food diary

ID:	Day of week:		Date:	
Time	**Type of eating***	**Description of food eaten and fluid drunk**	**Where, with whom?**	**Feelings around time of eating**

* eg. meal, snack, binge, pick, overeat; indicate if any methods of weight loss used

maintain her weight in the normal weight range without using inappropriate ways of losing weight may have to be reinforced for many years, and that she may need support and help at intervals to maintain her resolve and her weight. With this support she will gain insight into her behaviour and learn to cope without relapsing into a disordered eating behaviour.

The nutritional management of patients with eating disorders

Because patients with eating disorders usually have disordered ideas about the nature of the foods they eat, or do not eat; and because one of the aims of treatment is to restore normal eating behaviour, a dietitian is an important member of the team. The dietitian helps the patient to learn about foods and their nutritional content, helps her develop a normal attitude to food and to establish an appropriate eating behaviour to control the eating disorder, which will help her to recover from her eating disorder.

The dietitian takes a dietary history, which includes determining the patient's eating behaviours (it helps to use a food diary for a few weeks) and the foods avoided or chosen and why. The dietitian also explores the patient's past eating behaviours and weight changes if this has not already been done by the therapist.

The dietitian provides the patient with accurate information about basic nutritional matters (as many patients have quite erroneous beliefs about food and weight control) and how she can maintain weight in the desirable range for her.

With the information obtained by the therapist, the dietitian and other team members develop strategies to help anorexia nervosa patients restore their weight to the normal range and to maintain their weight in this range; to help bulimia nervosa patients to stop eating chaotically; and to help obese patients to develop ways of reducing their weight. In all cases the long-term aim is to help the person learn 'normal' eating behaviour.

The psychological treatment of eating disorders

Of the various psychological treatments proposed, one of them, *cognitive-behavioural therapy*, has given superior results in the first 2 to 3 months. After 12 months other treatments are equally as effective. Seldom is only one type of psychological treatment employed by therapists and most patients experience a more eclectic management of their eating disorder and related problems. This individualized, more flexible approach includes cognitive-behavioural therapy, interpersonal therapy, behaviour therapy, supportive psychotherapy, and nutritional therapy. This eclectic approach to treatment is beginning to produce superior results, possibly as it provides therapeutic interventions, that are relevant and appropriate for a woman at different stages of her treatment and recovery, and can be modified to fit in with her daily living and life events. Common sense suggests treating eating-related behaviour and thoughts and not the psychosocial factors associated with maintaining the eating disorder, or vice versa, would have a poorer long-term outcome.

Cognitive-behavioural therapy

This therapy is based on the concept that if you are provided with accurate information and develop a trusting relationship with your therapist, you can be persuaded to think differently (the cognitive part of the treatment) and will probably change your behaviour. In the treatment of eating disorders the therapy seeks:

(1) to explore the patient's thoughts and beliefs which maintain binge-eating and dangerous methods of weight control;

(2) to establish healthy eating habits;

(3) to establish regular eating behaviour, in which she eats three meals a day with one or two snacks if she desires;

(4) to help the patient learn about food, eating, shape, and weight, and to eliminate myths about food and eating;

(5) to help the patient increase her self-esteem and decrease the importance of her physical appearance in her evaluation of herself.

The patient and her therapist meet once or twice each week for three to five months. More details are shown in Table 29 (see p. 212).

This therapy seems to be especially effective in patients who have the binge-eating disorder or bulimia nervosa and to a lesser extent anorexia nervosa. Anorexia nervosa patients tend to maintain a rigid set of beliefs about weight and eating. They equate their self-esteem with their body shape and weight, that is, body shape and weight are the most important means by which they evaluate themselves. These two matters occupy most of their thoughts during the day and strongly influence their eating behaviour. Their rigidity of thought makes change harder to achieve.

Bulimic patients are also concerned about body shape and weight, and diet intermittently. They have a compulsion to binge-eat at frequent intervals. As they do not wish to become fat and know that the amount of food eaten during a binge will result in weight gain, they adopt various strategies, such as inducing vomiting or abusing laxatives, to prevent this.

Cognitive-behavioural therapy seeks to change these obsessional thoughts and behaviours so that the woman gains control over her eating and establishes a pattern of regular eating. This is achieved in several ways. In the first stage of the therapy, many therapists ask the patient to list what she perceives as the advantages and disadvantages of her eating behaviour. She and the therapist then explore and explain the disadvantages of the behaviour, as the patient perceives them, and discuss any distressing symptoms the patient may have.

With this information the therapist helps the patient develop ways of managing her eating and weight behaviours by changing her attitudes to them. During this time any erroneous beliefs about foods the patient may have (for example, beliefs about 'good' foods and 'bad' foods) are discussed.

Concurrently the patient meets with the dietitian to discuss dieting, the regulation of body weight, and dangerous methods of weight control.

In the second stage of the programme the patient is helped to talk about her feelings about her body and about food. She is helped to change negative feelings and to enhance her self-esteem, making body shape and weight less important to how she evaluates herself.

In some instances the involvement of the patient's partner or family may be suggested so that their attitudes and behaviours will not delay the patient's recovery or lead to a relapse after treatment.

Supportive psychotherapy

This technique is used to help a person who has a short-term crisis caused either by social problems or the illness itself. The person is encouraged to talk about her or his problems with a therapist who takes the person's worries seriously, who listens carefully and shows the patient that she is listening. The therapist provides reassurance, advice, and encourages the patient to take responsibility for changing her behaviour. This approach helps the woman learn to cope with stressful events without relapsing into her old behaviours.

Behaviour therapy

Under this treatment the therapist attempts to induce the patient to modify or to change her behaviour, by providing rewards or privileges, so that she learns to eat normally (see pages 226–7). For example, if a patient who has anorexia nervosa gains weight, or if a patient with bulimia reduces the frequency of self-induced vomiting, or if the obese person loses weight, a reward is given.

In the past the behavioural therapy programme was rigid and strict. For example, a patient who had anorexia nervosa was confined to bed, her personal possessions were removed and she was kept relatively isolated. As she gained a set amount of weight, she was given back her possessions, one at a time, and 'earned' other rewards, finally being allowed to get out of bed.

This punitive regimen has been replaced by a more flexible and lenient programme with much better results. In this programme rewards are given which may be as simple as praise for an achievement such as completing a task or modifying a behaviour.

The more lenient version of the treatment does not involve confinement to bed, provided the patient is making progress and participates in all the activities which have been arranged for her and the other eating disorder patients. If she feels that she is unable to join in these structured activities, she may be asked to rest in bed when no structured activities are taking place.

Interpersonal therapy

We noted (page 50) that a few eating disorder sufferers also have a personality disorder. Some psychiatrists have observed that cognitive-behavioural therapy, although effective in the short term, may not absolutely resolve the person's eating behaviours, particularly if the woman has a personality disorder. These psychiatrists believe that *interpersonal therapy* may help. This therapy aims to help the patient resolve interpersonal problems, such as unrealistic dependence on, idealization of, or hatred of a parent. It may also help women who have intrapersonal problems such as impulsive behaviour, lack of control over anger, and fluctuating moods.

The therapy is conducted by a sympathetic, supportive, undemanding therapist whom the patient feels she can trust. It consists largely of the therapist listening sympathetically as the patient recounts her feelings and expands on her perceived and submerged problems. This therapeutic approach, for the treatment of bulimia, has been shown by researchers in the UK and USA to be as effective as cognitive-behavioural therapy in the long term.

Disordered eating and compulsive exercising

Regular enjoyable exercise is beneficial to the health of all people and is particularly useful in helping obese people, who embark on a weight reduction programme to continue to lose weight (see page 263). A number of women who have one of the other eating disorders use exercise, not as a way of keeping fit but as a way of losing weight. They become compulsive exercisers. They may exercise compulsively during the time that they have anorexia nervosa or bulimia nervosa, and on recovering from these disorders may continue to exercise compulsively. In other words they replace their eating disorder with an 'exercise disorder'.

One such woman is Belinda. Belinda had bulimia nervosa. As she became free from her preoccupation with food and weight control, her eating habits returned to normal. For the past three years she has maintained a BMI of 22, and is happy with her appearance. But she is a compulsive exerciser.

Belinda wrote:

Each day of my life I try and fit my day around at least one session of quite strenuous, routine exercising—usually either 20 laps of a 50 metre pool or a 45 minute strenuous aerobic workout. If I cannot fit in my usual daily piece of exercise I feel guilty, worried, and up to a point anxious. Exercise has become an important part of my life. I should say that the main reason I exercise is for the actual feeling of being fit and feeling relaxed, not because I want to lose weight or look thin. I like me as I am now.

I do have the will-power to reduce exercising to only one session a day but I itch to keep pushing myself to it, even if my body just wants to flop. So I drive myself to do it and afterwards I feel really happy that I had pushed myself to do it, even though I didn't enjoy doing it at the time. I feel so sick of it all but would feel so unhappy and insecure if I stopped altogether. When I am emotionally upset over something important to me, I punish my body even more severely and increase the exercise. I feel weakness and no strength during an exercise session but I cannot stop doing it. I feel that I couldn't cut out my exercising completely but I am a strong-willed person and I feel positive about being able to live with myself if I reduce the intensity gradually. My aim is to keep doing three or four classes of aerobic exercise each week and have the occasional swim. Exercise used to be a really enjoyable feeling for me—now it is an addiction.

A woman who has Belinda's problem needs continued support and the chance to talk to her therapist whenever she feels that she needs to, so that she can express her feelings about the amount of exercise she does and can be helped to reduce it to a level which she can control without relapsing into disordered eating.

Women who are suffering from an exercise disorder may be asked to complete a daily exercise diary. This may help them to understand why they are exercising excessively and change the amount of exercise undertaken.

The advantages of having an eating disorder

Women who have eating disorders may see advantages in continuing with 'abnormal' eating behaviour. The advantages may be perceived by the woman as being greater than the disadvantages of the disorder, so that she is more comfortable persisting with the behaviour than changing it. The advantages vary and depend on whether the person has anorexia nervosa, has bulimia, or is severely obese.

An eating disorder may become an all-absorbing hobby and lead to the exclusion of most other age-related activities. In this way the sufferer is able to avoid making decisions and can reduce the challenges made or her. If the challenges are sexual, the woman may use her emaciation, or her obesity, to avoid them, claiming that her distorted body shape would repel rather than attract men. One of our patients said 'when my body weight is normal I am scared of people's expectations of me, and have to resist men who make advances. But when I am fat, I am able to avoid these problems'.

Other patients find that their emaciation, or obesity, makes other members of the family concerned. The woman becomes the centre of concern and induces the family to make expressions of love and to go to great lengths to 'look after her'. In this way she may be able to manipulate the family and obtains satisfaction from her behaviour. Other women manipulate close relatives by adopting 'illness

Table 19. Exercise diary

ID:	Date commenced:				
Day and time	Description of exercise or activity	Duration (mins)	Intensity mild, moderate, intense, very intense	Reason feel better, fitness, training, 'burn up energy'	Mood and feelings

* eg. meal, snack, binge, pick, overeat; indicate if any methods of weight loss used

behaviour'. Because the woman is perceived by her relatives as being 'ill' she is looked after. She is able to feel dependent, without feeling guilty, and may use this 'illness' to avoid a social or a family situation. For example, one of our patients lost weight each year in November and December so that she could be admitted to hospital for Christmas rather than having to spend it with her family. Another patient used her illness to justify her behaviour towards her husband, saying that 'my husband knew that he was marrying a sick person. If I get better he may not like me and we may separate'. By being ill she forced her husband to concentrate on her needs to the exclusion of his needs.

In other cases the person uses her eating disorder to avoid discussion of other problems in her relationship with her husband or family, or to avoid going out to social functions, at which she is uncomfortable. The person's emaciation or obesity may be used as an excuse to avoid competition. One of our patients ceased competitive swimming at the age of 12 and began putting on weight. By the time she was 19 her weight had risen to 108 kg (238 lbs, 17 st). She wrote:

> All the girls were too competitive. I'm out of that now, and can get on with everyone. When I was swimming people picked on me if I didn't do as well as they expected me to have done. Now I can do what I like, and do the things I like well. Now I'm fat, I find that people come and talk to me. They can see I have a problem. They can see I have a weakness of character, or I wouldn't eat so much. They have problems too. Other people can't see their problems, but as my problem is obvious they feel comfortable with me.

Another of our patients wrote about her eating disorder:

> I feel I have always needed the food to give me 'the rush' to make me high and happy. I know I use it as a protection barrier against experiencing and expressing emotional feeling with others and against physical and mental intimacy with a man. I have the need to break down this barrier and take charge of my life. You asked me what did I think would change if I lost the weight. I don't think the actual weight loss (or gain) would change anything, but if I could cease to look upon myself as a compulsive eater and feel relaxed about my food intake, then I feel I could tap the vitality and creativity that has eluded me all my life—I would feel I was functioning as a whole and not the several personalities I feel I am.

Obesity may also be a camouflage in families who are overweight. Being fat enables the person to fit in with the family and to behave as they do.

Some women feel a sense of achievement in being able to reduce their weight so that they become emaciated. One of our patients, aged 20, who had anorexia nervosa and who had, in her words, 'done nothing with my life' wrote to us saying 'At least I've done one thing well. I enjoy being my Doctor's worst patient.'

Most people have an idealized view of how they should appear: they want to be socially attractive, happy and outgoing, and popular. When the person realizes that she cannot achieve her ideal, she may adopt disordered eating behaviour, either losing weight and becoming thin or gaining weight and becoming obese. In this way she has an excuse which explains why she can't achieve her ideal. But at these extremes of weight she looks in a mirror and doesn't like her body image. She then tries to return to the normal weight range, by dieting and other methods.

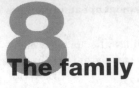

8
The family

It is really important to make time for yourself and for the other members of the family. This illness is extremely selfish and destructive and can cause a state of perpetual fear and exhaustion.

A side effect of the illness is that it shines a torch very brightly on the family's communication and coping skills.

Family support meetings are a wonderful opportunity to meet with other parents and discuss our feelings and concerns. It gives the parents a chance to 'have their say' and to listen to the experiences and frustrations of other parents in a similar situation.

Discovering your partner or a member of the family has an eating disorder can release a multitude of thoughts and questions. Some people have knowledge of the disorders either because a family member has already suffered or because they themselves are sufferers. When one mother discovered her daughter was suffering from anorexia nervosa she wrote this simple and loving letter to her daughter. In this letter she disclosed her own eating disorder.

Dear Georgina,

I hope I don't upset you too much by writing this letter. I only want to explain what will happen to your body if you don't eat. Please read on, as you're my daughter, I love you to bits and I don't want to lose you to anorexia nervosa.

I went through this terrible disease, I nearly died. The critic that talks to you in your head, making you feel so guilty for eating is so tormenting. You feel like committing suicide.

This disease controls your life. This critic or your subconscious (which is part of your mind which is not fully conscious but influences actions) in your mind telling you not to eat, it wants you to get thinner and thinner. It doesn't matter how much weight you loose your subconscious or critic in your mind will never be happy until you loose so much weight it will be life threatening. You won't be able to think clearly, make clear decisions, you'll always be angry with people. This subconscious will worry you so much it will drag you down, you'll stop having fun and you won't want to live. I thought about committing suicide several times when I was trying to cope with anorexia, as the worry to make a decision to eat, and then when you do eat something, it doesn't matter how small it is, this subconscious comes on full force making you feel so guilty that I thought it would be easy just to end it all. So I know how hard it is to make yourself eat. I understand fully what you are going through. What happens to your body when you don't eat? It slowly stops living.

Your periods stop.

Your bowels stop.

Your organs e.g. heart, lungs, kidneys are slowing down, then they'll stop.

Your body is dying slowly.

Your body is made up of living cells. These cells make up your organs, blood, bones, skin, etc. Your body needs food which has the nutrients to feed these cells. Every few days your living cells die off, but rebuild themselves with the food you eat. If you don't eat your cells won't rebuild. Your brain loses brain cells so you can't think clearly, people with this disease can start to steal from other people, as they aren't thinking clearly. Then they end up in court, trying to defend themselves. It happened to me.

So tell this critic or subconscious that you are going to eat, take one day at a time, don't think about tomorrow or next week. Think about how you'll get through today. Eat and then think well I got through today. Then when you wake up the next morning start the day off fresh again.

The reason you overeat when you start eating is your body needs the nutrients in the food, so when you start eating you can't stop because your body is saying 'I need more of this food to rebuild my cells'. This is when your subconscious comes in full force because you went against it and ate so you've made it very angry. Tell it to go to hell!

Let me explain it this way and I am not being funny, but you may understand it better. When you did something that made your father angry, when you went against his beliefs, he yelled and screamed and showed you he was angry even though you knew you were in the right, so you went ahead and did what you thought was right anyway.

Pretend your subconscious is like your father. It yells and screams, gets angry when you eat and go against its beliefs. But you know it's right to eat, so do what is right. Each time you went against your father's beliefs he got angry but you went ahead and did what you thought was right. In the end he gave up. You had won. Your subconscious is doing exactly the same thing. So if you start eating it will eventually give up and you will have won. The subconscious or critic is going to get very angry because you've eaten and it stays around in your mind reminding you not to eat, making you feel guilty. So when you eat it throws more guilt on you just like your Dad.

So fight it Georgina . . .

Love you always, Mum

A few months later her mother finished a letter to Georgina with the following:

. . . and the severe mental irritation and torment will slowly disappear. You've got to get to the stage Georgina, where you control Anorexia instead of Anorexia controlling you. I control my Anorexia. Anorexia is still controlling you and Anorexia will not be happy until it kills you, so to survive you have to learn to control Anorexia. You choose, it's your life.

Love, your Mum

The slow insidious onset of eating disorders and the impact of an eating disorder on the individual members of a family can be devastating. The sufferer becomes the focus of everyones' attention and energy. Other siblings can feel neglected and uncared for by their parents. Parents can become physically and mentally exhausted taking the sufferer for assessment and treatment, participating in the treatment, and trying to understand the illness and their daughter's behaviour. The slowness of the onset of eating disorders and sufferers' denial of their illness until they are seriously ill, all contribute to the failure of people to receive help early in their illness.

Cara is the mother of an 18-year-old, attractive student suffering from anorexia nervosa. She talked of her experiences:

I feel so helpless and I cannot understand it. What she says is alien to common sense. She looks like my daughter but what comes out of her mouth is foreign. It is as though a stranger has taken over her mind. She was a sensitive and commonsense girl, although she always has to be the best at everything she does. She is head girl at her school and is very popular. It amazed me when she confided she felt unsure of herself and hopeless at everything.

I blame myself for not recognizing her problem and seeking help for her earlier. I have always had the opposite problem as I am obese and did not realize what a terrible illness anorexia is. I thought people were lucky to be anorexic. She would bamboozle me with science and I would believe what she was telling me about food and the body as she was doing biology. The family had noticed she had lost weight and that she had become irritable, isolative, and moody. I thought it was just because she was working so hard for her final exams. Halfway though the year she asked us if she could change schools and then confessed that it was because she had an eating disorder, her friends were noticing and had told her she needed help. She had collapsed at school and barely eaten anything for two weeks. Once she had told us it was worse at home because then she could then eat less in front of us and eat only the food she prepared. She begged us not to take her to the doctors and that she would eat and she would show us she was all right. She did eat well, but selectively, in front of the family and so we allowed her to go away on holidays with her brother and my sister's family. She ate a lot. My sister told me she was eating more than the rest of the kids. By the end of the holiday she was very thin. She confessed to vomiting on the holiday. I took her to the family doctor who referred her to a specialist in eating disorders. She said she would go but only once so we could be told that there was nothing wrong. The doctor and the dietitian were very good and very pleasant and very thorough. Afterwards she told me they did not know what they were talking about, that she had just told them what they wanted to hear and was certainly not going to hospital to be treated and not going back to see them again. The specialist had made another time for me to go back to talk with her, even if my daughter would not come. She also explained about the hospital, gave us the address so we could talk to people at the hospital and gave me her phone number. To placate me my daughter told me she would eat all her meals at home, sit with us after the meal and visit the family doctor every week. She just wanted one more chance to show she would do it.

My sister rang me and asked what I was waiting for, was I waiting for her to die? I got such a shock. My sister and I went to her room and told her to pack her bags and that she was going to hospital. She cried and yelled and screamed 'you don't know what you are doing to me', 'you're humiliating me', you're taking away my choices', 'you can't make me', 'you don't understand', 'I'll die in hospital', 'nobody understands', 'I don't need food I'm different'. Her father who is always very soft with her told her she was going to hospital.

I had mixed emotions about leaving her in hospital; I was afraid she would run away, that I had betrayed her, that I had abandoned her, that she would never forgive me although I had no choice. Some of her ideas about food and eating seemed so weird I had thoughts of madness, something more had to be wrong not just an eating disorder.

Two months later:

I have my daughter back again. She looks and sounds like my daughter. There is still a along way to go. It is not over. She is eating and following the menu plan suggested by the hospital. She still makes no secret of her desire to be thinner but she says she will eat until after her exams.

There are a number of common questions parents and partners wish to have answered

- What causes the illness?
- What do you do to make her better?
- How can we help her?
- Should we comment on her eating and weight?
- Should you say anything when her behaviour is unacceptable?
- Why can't she eat?
- Why can't she stop eating?
- Will she ever get better or will she always have an eating disorder?
- How long will she need treatment?
- Will her bones recover?
- Will her heart and kidneys be permanently damaged?
- Has the family caused the eating disorder?
- Is it genetic?
- Will she be able to have children?
- Is it because her grandmother suffered depression?
- Will she ever be her old self again?
- Do you ever really recover from an eating disorder?

We have attempted to answer these as fully as possible in this book. It is not easy to give definitive answers to many questions as each person is unique and has different problems, experiences, and needs.

One mother, who has lived with and survived the suffering of two daughters with anorexia nervosa, prepared the following tips for parents to help them through the difficult times.

A parent's perspective

Tip: Fight the illness not the person

I believe that I was very fortunate that right from the very beginning of my experience with Anorexia Nervosa, I was able to understand that my daughters really had an illness. This enabled me to mobilise my energy and resources to fight the illness, rather than squabble with my daughters about their behaviours and other matters.

Tip: Don't blame yourself for causing the illness

No parent is ever going to do a perfect job, so I feel very sad when I observe parents going through a lot of anguish and guilt about doing something wrong that may have led their daughter to get an Eating Disorder. I consider myself very fortunate that in both instances I always felt that I was a good parent, and managed to retain my confidence in this matter.

When my elder daughter was sick, the head teacher of her school said to me 'Doesn't Anorexia Nervosa have something to do with an over-controlling mother?' This statement both upset and confused me, but wisely I ended up rejecting it.

Tip: Get professional help as quickly as possible

You are absolutely living in a fool's paradise if you believe that you don't need some professional help to get better, and I really urge you to seek help as quickly as you can. Try and find some health professionals with expertise/experience/interest in the illness, and if you have trouble locating the right health professional, then seek help from the Eating Disorders Association in your state.

I was totally shocked at the rapid progression of my younger daughter's illness, and it served a very valuable lesson to see how quickly things can sometimes deteriorate. It is important to be consistent and follow up with treatments, which can often take place over a long period of time.

Tip: Try to normalise family life

This is a really hard thing to do, as the illness plays havoc with the social fabric and functioning of the family. It is so easy to totally focus on only the ill person, and in the meantime family life can be disintegrating around one. It is sensible to try and get extra help and support for the family by confiding in other family members and close friends, attending family support groups, participating in family relationship counselling or family therapy when required.

Tip: Educate yourself about the illness

When my first daughter was ill there was very little information available about Eating Disorders, and so I went right through that whole experience never really knowing anything much about the illness. That was a really dreadful and frightening experience! Even when my second daughter was sick, I was still a bit slow seeking out information. I think it is much better to know the facts, so you have a good understanding of what you are dealing with, and a proper understanding of the health risks of the illness. Then you can make decisions about treatments and other matters concerning the health and welfare of your loved one, that are soundly based.

Tip: Give unconditional love and support

Giving unconditional love and support to the sick family member is a great gift to give to that person. Both of my daughters have since thanked me for giving them this gift, and I believe from the bottom of my heart that it assisted them greatly at the time. I think the 'giving' helped to maintain a healthy and close relationship that is still shared today. Bravo!!!

Tip: Try not to be too secretive about the illness

This is another really hard thing to do, as there is a natural tendency to want to protect the privacy of the family. When my first daughter was ill, I hardly told a soul, and looking back now, I can see just how isolated the poor family was, struggling to manage this illness so secretly. When you follow the secretive approach then you rob yourself of the practical and emotional support that can come from a more open discussion with others. There is obviously a balance that each individual person will need to find to satisfy his/her own individual needs.

Tip: Try to keep your sense of humour

This may sound a little bizarre when you are out there struggling with a terrible illness, but I believe a lot of good can come from fostering a positive attitude and environment. Try and make a conscious effort to do some enjoyable things together as a family, and don't feel guilty about enjoying life now and again. One of the most beautiful things I have ever heard was my daughter giggling with one of her friends after she came out of hospital. Somehow I thought I may never hear it again, and when I did, I knew she was getting better—it made me so happy, and gave me so much hope for her future!

Tip: Give respect to the person with the illness

Once you are able to acknowledge that an Eating Disorder is an illness, then the person with the illness is entitled to a level of respect for the suffering he/she is encountering. It can take a great deal of personal courage for the person with the illness to take the necessary steps and follow the treatments that are a part of the recovery process.

Tip: Sometimes you may need to be firm

This can be another of those really hard things to do, but there are times when a loving firmness is needed. Sometimes the sick family members may be irrational about a matter, and it is important to show a consistency in behaviour that always puts their best health first. Sometimes this can take quite a surprising amount of personal courage too!

I shall conclude with a poem I wrote about my younger daughter, when I first realised she was making progress, and I could glimpse again the emergence of her beautiful personality.

The blossom opens

The blossom opens
And slowly turns towards the sun,
Its warming rays to kiss,
The sun brings hope and life.
The emerging flower is beautiful,
With petals still fragile
And fragrance sweet,
And morning dew glistening
On the opaque green leaf.

My daughter is this blossom,
And I watch in awe
As the blossom becomes a smile,
Fresh and open, so happy.
The dew becomes a cascade
Of tingling laughter.
My heart feels warm now,
Nature's cycle is complete

Anon 24 November 1996

Helen described her experience with the illness and recovery:

The realisation that your child is ill and seriously, is such a shock. I kept hoping it would just go away. To watch a beautiful, vital child decline into the walking dead is devastating. The feeling of helplessness and ineptitude was overwhelming. I kept thinking if I could be with her every waking moment I could encourage her, hold her, protect her from herself. I felt absolutely bereft. I mourned the child she had been. Sometimes I think I helped, other times I said it all wrong. I was walking a precipice and I felt so alone. I shut everyone out of our problem, because I was sure I could handle it and I knew how little things could plunge her into deep despair. I trusted no one, not even her father. I felt only I could help her. I took her to our family doctor and I suddenly knew we were not alone anymore. We started seeing a person who really understood about eating disorders.

It has been almost 2 years and it was very intense. Progress was slow at first and the threat of hospital was always very real. Bianca was angry a lot of the time and defensive, but that made me feel hopeful, because even at her worst she never allowed herself to be angry. She was always perfect. Some days she seemed to be making progress and then there would be weeks of depression, and worse a new development, she was shutting me out. But I knew however hurtful it was, it was also healthy. She was transferring her dependence onto her therapist. This was hard to deal with but I trusted her to protect the integrity of the family and especially my relationship with my daughter. So, slowly I felt a sense of myself re-emerging. After being totally consumed in another being I could experience longer and longer periods of time not thinking about her. We stopped being the centre of each other's world. A new sense of peace developed it was bliss.

Of course Bianca put on weight and looked beautiful and she was laughing again, and starting to see friends. She got a job and really came out of herself. When she started going out we were so thrilled.

When she was ill she was always acting. Acting happy, acting interested, acting friendly. Now she has a real life. Not always easy or happy, but real. Before she was caricature of herself. Now she is whole with all the complexities of a wonderful healthy teenager. She has a boyfriend, lots of friends and a life full of colour. Her self-confidence is growing in leaps and bounds. She's less and less afraid of being herself, less and less afraid people won't like her.

As a mum my role in Bianca's life has been a roller-coaster ride. There was a long time that I felt really bad about myself and what a failure I was. How could a beautiful, happy and loved little girl want to disappear? It had to be us who let her down, who failed to give her self-esteem. I took total responsibility and it nearly killed me too. But now I feel better about myself, and even proud of the role I played in Bianca's recovery. There are times I feel totally left out and a bit nervous about where she is in her head, but she has grown so much. She has lived a lifetime in the last 2 years. And knows herself in a way that usually only comes with age. I trust her intuition about many things, but especially about her own needs.

9
Anorexia nervosa

I just wish that anorexia would get the blazes out of my life! From 1982 to now, everything I do, have done or didn't do centres around my fear of food. For those of you not familiar with the demonic workings of anorexia—fear of food and getting fat are its basic elements.

The definition and diagnostic criteria for anorexia nervosa were discussed on page 26. These have been codified by the American Psychiatric Association and are shown in Table 5 (p. 26).

Anorexia nervosa affects women fifteen times more commonly than men and usually begins during adolescence or in early adulthood. It is unusual for the illness to occur for the first time after the age of 45, and if it does, the eating disorder is usually associated with other mental or physical problems.

Anorexia nervosa seems to be occurring more frequently among young women in the developed countries but is also being reported in countries in the less developed world. In the former countries the illness affects at least one woman aged 13–25 in every thousand, reaching a peak incidence of one in 200 among adolescent girls aged 14 to 18.

A few children under the age of 13 also develop anorexia nervosa. In spite of media hype, anorexia nervosa is not occurring in epidemic proportions.

Gwyneth describes her experience:

Over the past three years of my life I have struggled and fought a vicious and simply destructive disease. Anorexia nervosa. During this period of my life, it not only destroyed my body and soul, it took every aspect of my social life, family, friends, and relatives down with it too. My will to live and the very concept of how to live life was lost. I lived each day waiting for the next to come, moving from one 'supposed' meal to the next. My life was ruled by food (or the lack of) and food made the rules for my life.

Two years ago I was on a holiday on a tropical Island and I wrote in my diary *'I can't wait until each day is over, I rush to bed in case I get hungry and feel like eating. I can't control things away from home, the food is different and I'm ruining everyone's holiday. I have decided to stop fighting Anorexia and give it my life to make everyone else's happier without the stress of me. Mum said she just wants me to be happy and that's what I've chosen to do for her.'*

When I look back at the insanity of things I wrote, I can finally understand how twisted and blinded the starving mind can become. When suicide is the only answer I saw, I thank God that something deep inside told me I was wrong. This is when I needed the help of others to show me the answers I couldn't find alone.

Although it has been a slow and painful process I have finally reached the once 'unattainable' recovery, that I thought you only read about in books. One by one, the ridiculous rituals and lists of rules I had set for myself (in order to control my body and life) were literally crossed out. From never using moisturisers on my body (for fear that the fats would seep through my skin) to overloading foods with chilli, I gradually learned to let go of these habits and ironically found I was getting a greater sense of control over myself.

With each change I saw in my personality as I slowly put on 0.5 kg by 0.5 kg, I gained more hope and determination. Don't get me wrong, there were many times I slipped backwards, but I persisted and am reaping endless benefits now having put back on almost 10 kilograms.

Within a month of reaching my set 'goal' weight that had been determined for me by the professor, I had my period back, my depressions ceased, I developed breasts and the figure a woman of 18 should appear to have, a boyfriend, a social life, basically normal eating and exercising habits, and most importantly, confidence and respect for myself. Something I had not known for a very long time.

There was definitely an extreme separation that occurred between myself and my mother too (but a healthy one), simply due to the fact that I had depended on her so heavily during my illness and all of a sudden I was on my own again. This has been one of the hardest things for both her and I to accept and learn to deal with. What I realise now is that it is not only I that has to forget old habits but my family does too. Mum was so used to monitoring my food intake, mood, and exercise that she had to forcibly distance herself and hand back to me the responsibility of my health and life.

There is always that constant fear of losing myself to anorexia again, but I know what keeps me strong is remembering the changes that I have seen in my life and me as I have fought my way to recovery. I have never been happier. I am building myself a career, I'm healthy and fit, I am in complete love with my boyfriend whom I have been with for almost a year now, the tension and stress my family felt each day is completely gone (bar the odd 'she's taken my shoes again' saga). My friends have the 'old me' back and I'm making the most of every day I live on this earth.

Victims of anorexia nervosa have different experiences.

Case history: Alison
Alison was a tall, slim girl, who at the age of 15 had begun dieting with the other members of her class at school. She did this to feel part of the group rather than because she needed to lose weight. She managed to stick to the diet better than most of her peers, her weight falling from 52 kg (115 lbs, 8st 3 lb; BMI 20.4) to 47 kg (104 lbs, 7st 6 lbs; BMI 18.4). 'I was able to keep to the diet because my family are health freaks, and I began to feel guilty if I ate "bad fattening" foods.' About this time she began to be teased by the other girls about her small breasts and became self-conscious about them and her bottom, which she said 'stuck out too much'.

Alison was ambitious and wanted to do well at school. In her last two years she seldom went out to social events, because she felt she had to study, which she did conscientiously. 'Perhaps I was rather obsessional about study', she said, 'but I wanted to do well'. As well as studying hard, she cooked for the family, making cakes and biscuits (which she avoided eating) in addition to cooking the main meals. She perceived her household duties as helping her mother, who had a full time job, but her sister perceived them as trying to be a 'goody goody'.

She passed her school examinations and enrolled in a catering course because she enjoyed the practical aspects of cooking and preparing food. About this time she began to weigh herself each day, and continued to diet so that she became thinner. Her sister left home, and told Alison that in her opinion she had only 'lost weight to get all the attention of the family and put her sister's nose out of joint'. The sibling rivalry was marked.

Over the next two years, Alison continued with her course and proved an outstanding student. During this period her father's weight

Case history: Alison (continued)

increased by about 14 kg (31 lbs, 2 st 3 lbs) whilst his daughter's weight continued to decline, so that at graduation Alison weighed 32 kg (70 lbs, 5st; BMI 12.6). Her father was diagnosed as having a high blood pressure and instructed to lose weight which he found difficult to do. Alison tried to help, informing him what to eat, and worked out diets for him, 'counting the calories' of the food in the diets she devised.

She recognized that she was very thin and that she no longer menstruated, but she felt she was eating as much as other people, and if she are more she would 'put on weight rapidly and become fat'. She felt safe as long as her weight did not increase. She also felt it was wrong to eat more than others when 'there were so many starving people in the world'.

When she was 19 she visited a doctor about constipation which worried her and which she did not connect with her small intake of food. She was diagnosed as having anorexia nervosa and admitted to hospital for refeeding which was not successful. She responded to out-patient treatment and over seven months her weight increased to 44 kg (97 lbs, 6 st 13 lbs; BMI 17.3). She wanted to put on more weight but was worried that if she did she 'would lose control and become fat'. With persuasion and persistence she was induced to gain weight and by the age of 20 had stabilized at 49 kg (108 lbs, 7 st 10 lbs; BMI 19.2). She now believed that if her weight increased to 50 kg (110 lbs, 7 st 12 lbs; BMI 19.6) she would 'lose control', but was happy to keep it at about 49 kg.

At this time she moved to a city 125 miles away to run a restaurant, and began to write letters.

Two months after her move she wrote:

Well, I weighed myself recently and I'm just 47 kg (104 lbs, 7 st 6 lbs). I'm not consciously trying to lose weight, but its obvious I'm not eating enough. I'm not missing out on any meals and eat a varied diet—including supposedly fattening foods. But my brain still ticks in the same way as before—that I'm not allowed to get fat. What's wrong with me? I can't go through life needing someone to reinforce the fact that I have to be at a higher weight before my hormones will start functioning. I still feel the need to be reassured that it's OK to be 52 or 54 kg (115 lbs or 119 lbs, 8–8$\frac{1}{2}$ st)—whatever I'm supposed to be. Now it's only me, telling me I'm not allowed to get fat. I can't believe I'm so thick headed!

Case history: Alison (continued)
Two months later:

One positive fact is that I haven't lost any weight. But how true that at a low weight, your moods are more erratic and depressed and mental functioning is impaired. I can't believe it—people keep telling me I don't eat enough but the whole day is 'a meal'. I can't stuff anymore into me. If my bowels would function normally may be I would have more appetite. I've been more tense in the last 3 or 4 weeks, it upsets me terribly. The more depressed I become the less I want to be with people. I could quite happily exist alone—I'm constantly accusing myself of things and apologizing to other people. I talk to other people but do not listen to what they say. I know I must be a pain but I can't seem to do anything about it. I don't want to come back because I know I would run home to the family for protection—they'd assure me that everything was OK when I know damn well it isn't. I'm wasting my life—it is a chore just to get through the day. I want to come back and talk to you when I get my holidays later this year. Three months after her last letter, Alison returned to the Clinic. She was neatly, even elegantly, dressed but look thin. Her BMI was 16. Over the next few months she increased her weight at the rate of 1 kg (2.2 lbs) a month and has now maintained a body weight of 50 kg (110 lbs, 7 st 12 lbs; BMI 19.6) for the past two years. She has formed relationships and has a steady boyfriend. She continues to excel in her work as manager of a restaurant.

Preoccupation with food and fear of gaining weight

The first of the diagnostic criteria for anorexia nervosa is that the sufferer has a fear of gaining weight and becoming fat. She embarks on a relentless pursuit of becoming or remaining thin. Food and its avoidance becomes an all-absorbing hobby to the exclusion of most of the other activities she would normally indulge in at that age, especially social occasions when food is usually present and eating expected. The preoccupation with weight is such that most patients can give a detailed history of their weight changes, including changes as small as 0.5 kg (1 lb) over periods as short as a week. The preoccupation about food and weight control and the overwhelming urge to become thin leads anorexia nervosa patients to use a range of eating behaviour to achieve their desire. Cassandra described her fear of fatness when her BMI was 15:

My arms are so flabby, my stomach huge, and I am really getting worried because lunch is coming up. I really wanted Mum to help me think I can eat it but she's gone now and I feel so sick I cannot face food.

I know I should have it but something deep inside me tells me not to—I really want to listen to it because I know it will help me feel better later—and help my problems (ie FATNESS!). I'm worried Mum is going to get me lunch or ask me what I want and I don't know whether. I'm hungry or not yet. I need someone to help me decide and understand. I feel very bad because I didn't go for a walk this morning and the fact that I have time to go now and haven't yet makes it even worse. I'm very tired and don't think I will go—but I know I'll be punished with FATNESS for that. I don't know why I don't avoid that consequence and go—but I really don't think I can.

I have been having very bad thoughts again and have wanted to die. Last night I took out a lot of laxatives and other fat stopping pills but Mum came into my room before I took them. They are in my box now—and I am worried I might take too many one day. I put the scales back in my room because I have to monitor my weight closely at the moment as I have lost a little weight yet I *know* I am fatter which is confusing me and so I think I should keep an eye on the scales to see what is happening to me.

Young women whose weight has usually been in the normal range before their eating disorder began generally lose weight by the simple method of eating less and by avoiding situations in which they have to eat. In order to avoid eating they make excuses such as 'I don't feel hungry at the moment so I'll eat some later' when told by parents that a meal is ready. Other excuses offered are 'I have eaten already'; 'I've decided to become vegetarian'; 'I have an allergy to . . . (certain foods)'; 'I feel sick'. The young women tend to avoid social occasions, and may lock themselves in their room and ask not to be disturbed. They may be competitive and are often obsessive about their work, which enables them to avoid social occasions where food is eaten. In addition to strict dieting, they may use exercise as a method of losing weight. This may involve jogging, playing squash, attending 'health farms', 'or working out' at a gymnasium for long hours.

Case history: Jennifer

Jenny was 15 when she went on holiday on her own. At the holiday resort she entered a beauty contest and came second. That night she got drunk for the first time and had her first experience of sexual intercourse. She felt guilty about being drunk and about having sex. At school she was a good student, worked hard, and excelled in sports, being in the school swimming, hockey, and basketball teams. On her return from holiday she believed that she would have won the beauty contest if she had been slimmer and if her thighs and bottom had been smaller. She decided to go on a diet to lose weight, and this resulted in arguments with her mother, who thought that Jennifer was already slim.

Jenny compromised by offering to do the cooking (in reality it was to help her have control over the calorie content). During meals she moved the food about the plate so that she appeared to be eating. She avoided cream and fatty foods, telling her family that they made her feel sick. She spent long hours alone in her room studying and in the evenings attended dancing classes. In her room she exercised strenuously, for 15 to 20 minutes every two hours, and played music to hide the noise of her exercises from her parents. She told them that the music helped her concentrate upon her studies. She became obsessional about her weight, weighing herself before and after meals, before and after bouts of exercise, and before and after going to the toilet.

At about this time she was chosen to represent her state in a folk-dancing championship and increased her daily exercise, telling her parents that she had to be 'super fit to help my team win'. With increasing exercise and a limited food intake, Jennifer's weight dropped from 53 kg (117 lbs, 8 st 5 lbs; BMI 22) to 45 kg (99 lbs, 7 st 1 lb; BMI 18.7). She wore loose clothes to disguise her low weight from her family. However, one morning her mother saw her naked and was horrified. Jenny promised to eat more, but again managed to disguise the amount she ate and whenever possible slipped food from her plate to the family dog.

As the time of the folk-dancing championships approached Jenny increased the amount of exercise she did daily, and, because she still felt she was too fat, restricted her food intake still further. Two weeks before the championships she collapsed and was admitted to hospital. Her weight was now 32 kg (70 lbs, 5 st; BMI 13.3). In hospital she felt that she was no longer in control of her weight, she became agitated, and was given antidepressant medication. With refeeding she gained 8 kg (17 lbs) and with her parents' agreement discharged herself from hospital.

At home she continued to exercise excessively and again collapsed. She was readmitted to hospital and remained in hospital until her weight

Case history: Jennifer (continued)
had increased to 51 kg (112 lbs, 8 st; BMI 19.3;). During this hospital admission she agreed to and worked out a menu plan with the dietitian. Since discharge she has maintained her weight at around 46 kg (108 lbs, 7 st 10 lbs; BMI 18.7). At first she was terrified that she would gain weight and began exercising again. This has become an obsession, so much so that she jogs in the streets if her doctor is running late with his appointments. However, in spite of a strenuous exercise programme, she eats sufficient food to maintain her body weight.

Binge-eating and potentially dangerous methods of weight control

The second group of anorexia nervosa patients, who have more often been overweight before the start of the illness, and whose weight tends to fluctuate during the illness, use potentially dangerous methods to lose weight. In this behaviour they resemble binge-eaters. They usually deny that they have any concern about their weight. In public, or among the family, they may appear to eat normal amounts of food. However, having eaten, they make excuses to leave the group and induce vomiting, and may combine this with the excessive use of laxatives. Because of their eating habits, phases of severe weight reduction, causing emaciation, are interspaced with periods of weight gain. They tend to be fairly social, and are less obsessional than the 'dieters'. In some cases, the woman has been a binge-eater for several months, or even years, before a decision to lose weight relentlessly precipitates her into anorexia nervosa.

Case history: Barbara
Barbara thinks that she began binge-eating when she was ten. The binge usually consisted of eating a packet or two of biscuits, several ice creams, and whatever she could find in the house when she came home from school. By the age of 13 years Barbara had begun to menstruate and weighed 70 kg (154 lbs, 11 st; BMI 28). In the following year she became interested in boys, became aware that she was fat, and stopped eating sweets and cakes. She knew she was overweight but was popular and had an active social life. As she was intelligent she achieved high grades at school. Over the next five years her weight decreased slowly

Case history: Barbara

so that by the age of 18 she weighed 63 kg (139 lbs, 9 st 13 lbs; BMI 25.5). At this time problems in her parents' marriage were becoming apparent. She obtained entry to university and enjoyed the experience, but at the end of the second year she decided that she must lose weight for the coming summer and began dieting. She also avoided eating whilst studying. As a result her weight fell to 57 kg (126 lbs, 9 st; BMI 23.1) over a period of four months She restricted her diet further, began counting calories, and started jogging. In addition she started taking laxatives daily because of constipation. Her parents had now separated and after trying to live with her father she moved into her mother's house. By winter her weight had dropped to 36 kg (80 lbs, 5 st 10 lbs; BMI 14.6) and her periods had ceased. She abused laxatives and on days of overeating took emetics so that she would vomit afterwards. She was also able to obtain diuretics from the family doctor for her 'fluid retention'. With these medications, the dieting, and the vomiting she became sufficiently ill to be admitted to hospital for refeeding. In hospital she lost control of her eating and ate everything she could obtain, with the result that her weight increased rapidly and she was praised by the staff. Her weight was now 46 kg (99 lbs, 7 st 1 lb; BMI 18.6) and she was discharged 'cured of anorexia nervosa'.

Her preoccupation with being extremely thin had ceased, but she still had an eating disorder. This became apparent later that year when she went to India with a group of students to visit Kashmir. She wrote to the clinic from there:

I spent the first 3 weeks of the holiday trekking in Kashmir which is astonishingly beautiful. I was enjoying the fantastic scenery, the fresh air, and the exercise and seemed to escape my problems up here high in the mountains. But on the last days of the trek, I got extremely sick with acute dysentery, fever—the works—and reached Srinagar in great distress doubled up by unbelievable cramps. I had to stay in bed for several weeks feeling pretty rotten. Four of my friends got hepatitis and the hospital was appalling. So what did I do? I ate, believe it or not! Few but ex(?) anorexics could eat with such gusto, in spite of abdominal pains, but somehow I managed and I have continued to eat since I came home. I am now even fatter than before—I'm 66 kg (145 lbs, 10 st 5 lbs) and still have diarrhoea and cramps at times. But these will go; the stool tests are negative. What I'm rather distressed about is my weight (what else!) as I feel it is slowly destroying my ability to cope with everyday life. Just as my eating behaviour is out of control, my life seems to be getting

Case history: Barbara (continued)
the same way. My social life is eventful and fun, on the whole, and I'm not withdrawn, but I have that frantic sense of imminent doom and I'm incredibly fearful of putting on more weight. I've tried many ways to overcome whatever it is that makes me eat but I can't break the pattern for more than 2 or 3 days. I've thought of the alternatives—getting fatter, vomiting, starving—even suicide . . . but actually I'd give my right arm to have the whole lot sorted out. I'm enjoying Uni, and the course which is full of interest (when I'm not occupying my mind with stagnant thoughts of weight and food). I'd rather anything than spending half my time (and all my money) on food. And it was this feeling that made me diet, and become anorexic, two years ago.

I am lying down listening to Mozart. I should be writing an essay but I ate so much yesterday that I have bad cramps plus an upper abdominal pain from eating too much today. Musing over how long it will take to lose 19 kg (42 lbs, 3 st) in the shortest quickest way—etcetera, etcetera—and it sure is a BLOODY WASTE of TIME. I've got a lovely family, some good friends, a fantastic boyfriend, lots of material assets—and instead I retreat into this awful life I've created for myself. Is it going to be like this forever? I couldn't stand it for much longer. I feel like it is moving in upon me and asphyxiating me. I can't get much done at all as I'm so caught up in this 'vicious circle'—I'm just as obsessed with food as I was 2 years ago and I want to escape or it will be 3 years, 4 years—ad infinitum. An unbearable thought.

Anorexia nervosa in males

Anorexia nervosa occurs in males fifteen times less frequently than in females. It begins in the same way, its clinical characteristics and its course are identical to that in females. Most males with anorexia nervosa spend hours each day jogging, bodybuilding, doing press-ups, and other exercises. They are as obsessed about food and body image as women and may become personal trainers or work in the food industry. Why males should pursue thinness so relentlessly is obscure, as adolescent men seek to be muscular rather than thin Unlike women, men do not experience a rapid unwanted increase in body weight in early adolescence or the accompanying loss of self-esteem.

It has been suggested that anorexia nervosa may be higher among homosexual men but this has not been confirmed and has not been reported in previous studies of men and eating disorders. Males suffering from anorexia nervosa are more likely to have additional problems including obsessive-compulsive disorder, alcohol and substance abuse, and personality disorder. Men who develop anorexia nervosa may also binge-eat; an example is John who explained why he binge-ate in a letter:

Whenever I get worried about the fact that I have anorexia nervosa and that I binge-eat as well (and I have to admit vomit after the binge) my thoughts turn to Uncle Harry and his character, personality, and his periods of depression. I don't know him too well so the following is only a theory but it seems to fit to our—his and my—personality traits and our mental histories. The theory came into my mind when I was talking to Bill about my eating problems; I don't talk to many people about them but I did to Bill. Bill said 'You set your standards pretty high'. He's right, of course, I do and it may explain my recent overconscientiousness and overconsciousness—an overconsciousness of myself which has trapped me in a small world of self so that I have found it hard to work, to study, to relax, to sleep, to concentrate or even to communicate with others. I have become overconscious of everything I say and do. So when Bill said 'you set your standards pretty high', at first I thought it sounded like flattery. But when I thought about it more I realized that it may have some truth in it.

I have to admit that prior to moving here I had a method of relaxing and releasing this tension. I'd binge. Certainly I felt guilty as I was a strain and burden on Mum and Dad. Since moving I have tried to have as few binges as possible. In all fairness, I have cut down on binges. (I try not to keep count, but I must maintain this positive attitude.) However, regardless of any physical success I *may* have had, the mental impact of telling myself 'I can't' and 'I must not' or 'I intend to go the next three weeks without a single binge', creates much tension and depression. Remember, I no longer have 'bingeing' as an outlet for any 'natural' everyday type tensions. As a matter of fact, the desire to *stop* bingeing has become a tension-maker within itself.

Case history
The result is that my tension and depression builds to the point of desperation when I feel I am near insanity and even

Case history (continued)

contemplate suicide. It never gets any further than this as (and I am sad to admit this, but it seems true) I end up having a binge. Somehow, I end up feeling more relaxed.

However, I then promise myself to make a more determined effort to beat the bingeing and the cycle starts again. This tension 'build-up' cycle not only applies to my bingeing. It also applies to other projects, plans, and aspects of my life. I seem to set a goal that *may* be just that little bit too high for me. I don't accept myself and my own limitations. I seem to set myself up for failure.

Everyone suffers tensions. Those who handle them best seem to have some way of relaxing. I *used* to have by bingeing. Although I still have binges *physically*, I now seem to have placed a *mental* prohibition on binges. The *mental* prohibition itself creates tension which sometimes cause a *physical* binge and thus not only becomes ineffective, but also becomes a causal factor itself.

In other words, I either have to find another method of relaxation or, at least for the time being, accept my human weaknesses and, by this, I mean accept an at least limited amount of bingeing. Two important points: first, another form of relaxation will probably have to come about naturally. I don't think I will be able to consciously search for one. If I try to search for one the mere fact that I am conscious of it can prevent relaxation. Second, I find it hard to mentally accept a limited amount of bingeing in the future. Both because I have become determined to defeat it (once again setting my goal too high??) and because of my insecurity, especially financially, as I no longer live with Mum and Dad. Although Mum and Dad have assured me that they would always help me (and I believe, trust, and love them) there is a large physical distance between us. I also fear that if I let up my 'guard' against bingeing to allow 'limited' bingeing (by limited I mean once, maybe twice, a week), I may end up slipping back and bingeing more. Would Mum and Dad help me then? . . .

Anyway, I digress. Uncle Harry is a person who sets high standards for himself. I don't feel I'm guessing. He's achieved a hell of a lot in his life; but instead of being proud of it, he is only

Case history (continued)

ashamed/guilty (for the want of better words) for what he hasn't achieved. Look!! He played first class cricket, he's been a successful headmaster. He's had a successful family life (many don't these days) and he's raised three healthy, intelligent, and successful children. He's retired from work and is just as well off as he was when he worked. (This might not be a fantastic achievement, but how many people can retire at 50 yrs. with the prospect of leading a secure, fulfilling, and useful life.) Me? I haven't achieved any of these things (and actually don't seem to have achieved much), except being thin.

Anyway, the key to Uncle Harry's and my problems is *tension*!! This tension isn't caused by external factors (such as family, work, or social problems) but internal standards we set ourselves. I seem to continually set myself up to fail by setting goals that are not within my reach (at least in the time span I allow and expect). It is probably about time we accept our own weaknesses (food may be mine but I'll never admit or accept it??), our inevitable failing, our limitations, and the limits of the human body and mind. We can only do our best and unfortunately our best may sometimes be less than what we, ourselves, expect. Don't worry about whether other people accept us—if they can't accept us as we are with our limitations, that's *their* problem, *not* ours . . .

Uncle Harry's and my basic problem is the self-inflicted tensions we impose on ourselves. In the past, I have used bingeing to relieve my tensions. I sometimes fear I may suffer nervous breakdowns if I can't find a way to relax. Just lately, especially with my at least attempted mental (if not physical) non-acceptance of bingeing, my fears of having some sort of breakdown have been far from a fantasy. Anyway, the answer for Uncle Harry and me may be this: *accept* ourselves for what we are; *accept* our limitations. For Uncle Harry this may be accepting that he was not meant to be some of the things he feels he should have been or had a duty to be or do. For me, this may mean accepting (and I still don't want to admit it) bingeing to a small extent while I allow some other element to replace it naturally (but by God, I'll still search hard and experiment until I find this other element).

Case history (continued)

I also have a great need for affiliation, friendship, love, and a need to feel needed. But as I said, if others can't accept us as we are, that's *their* problem. There will always be someone to accept us as we are (these people are friends worthy of having).

If we accept ourselves, we can relax. Tension and our inner self-competitiveness will float away. We can then concentrate on giving to others and the world, those good points we have *AND EVERYBODY* (no matter who they are) has good points!! *EVERYBODY!!!*

The onset of anorexia nervosa

Anyway, when I first started to diet I set myself a specific amount that I was allowed to eat each day—usually birdlike portions. I would suffer endlessly if my plan was disrupted by an invitation to lunch. To eat a large meal in the middle of the day was a source of a most guilty conscience for days after, that was the extent of my paranoia! I stuck to my diet religiously. But my reward was always a Coconut Honey Log on Friday afternoons, and I allowed myself to eat bread during the weekend.

The decision to diet in order to become thin is triggered in a variety of ways, depending on the woman's personality and the particular circumstances in which she finds herself. Often the onset of anorexia nervosa in a young girl follows an awareness that she does not like the shape or size of her body. As has been mentioned, concern about body shape and size is common among adolescent girls; but, in the case of those who have anorexia nervosa, it becomes an obsession. The young woman's preoccupation with her body and her weight often follows a challenge; for example, her family or her friends may tease her about her shape and her weight, or it may follow a competition with a friend to lose weight. Family stress may be a factor of considerable importance in triggering the onset of anorexia. The most common factor is an independence/dependence struggle between the young woman and one or both parents, who give mixed messages, for example, 'you must be independent but we need you at home'. In other cases the young woman is confused: wanting to be independent yet dependent. For example, she may say 'I want to do things my way but I want the security of home.' In other instances the onset of anorexia is associated with a series of events which are stressful in themselves, such as a break-up with a boyfriend, the first experience of sexual intercourse, an unwanted pregnancy, marriage, a major examination, or with a period of further deterioration in already stressful circumstances such as parents separating; or increasing pressure on the girl to 'achieve' at school in extra-curricular activities such as sport or dancing.

The effects of weight-loss behaviours

Before I started to lose weight I weighed about 52 kg (115 lbs, 8 st 3 lbs) and had reached my present height. Common sense tells me that my weight was not heavy for that height. But common sense had left me and I wanted to weigh about 43 kg (95 lbs, 6 st 11 lbs). And I achieved it! The strange thing is that whenever I went to buy new clothes I always saw how revoltingly thin my image in the mirror actually was. But I still felt fat.

Behaviours aimed at achieving weight loss, such as starvation, self-induced vomiting, the abuse of laxatives and enemas, diuretics, and excessive physical exercise may cause biochemical, psychological, and physical disturbances.

The biochemical changes associated with anorexia nervosa

Most of the psychological and physical changes are dependent on the biochemical changes which follow starvation, severe dieting, and dangerous methods of weight control. The main biochemical disturbances are dehydration and changes in the levels of some blood electrolytes (Fig. 13).

The sequence of these changes is shown in Fig. 13. Although this figure may seem rather complicated at first, it shows that if an anorexia nervosa sufferer starves herself, induces vomiting, abuses purgatives and diuretics, or indulges in excessive exercise, she may as a result develop a number of physical disturbances, the most serious being heart or kidney failure and death. In most cases the changes are less life-threatening but are nevertheless disturbing to the sufferer and to her family and relatives.

Starvation or severe dieting, purgative and diuretic abuse, and excessive exercise may lead to dehydration (and low blood potassium level). These are the underlying reasons for the psychological and physical symptoms which we discuss later.

Self-induced vomiting and dehydration may cause a metabolic alkalosis, in which the woman's blood becomes alkaline due to a loss of bicarbonate and a decrease of potassium and chloride. The metabolic alkalosis may impair the woman's neuromuscular function, so that she becomes easily fatigued, has muscle weakness, and may develop tingling in her hands and feet and involuntary hand clenching, which is very disturbing. More seriously the metabolic changes may lead to irregular heart-beats and occasionally to heart failure.

A few women who abuse laxatives develop a metabolic acidosis, because of loss of bicarbonate-rich fluid in the loose stools. This may

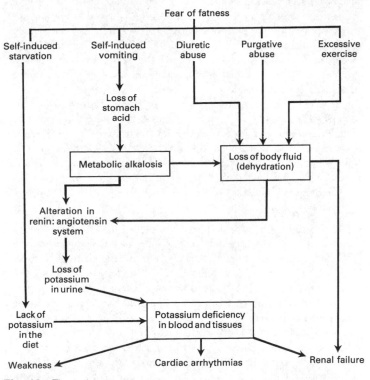

Fig. 13. Electrolyte problems in anorexia nervosa.

lead to hyperventilation (over-breathing) and high levels of chlorine in the blood, which very rarely causes heart failure.

In spite of the severity of the weight loss or the maintenance of a very low body weight, and in spite of the use of potentially dangerous methods of weight control, it is surprising how few sufferers develop potassium deficiency. In part this is because the body develops physiological compensatory mechanisms. In addition, many women who have anorexia nervosa are aware that their behaviours

Case history: Sandra

Sandra was a tall, quiet girl who was considerate, competent, and well-liked at school. In consequence she was given responsibility both at school and at home.

When she was 14 years old, her weight was 67 kg (148 lbs, 10 st 8 lbs; BMI 23.7). She felt that she was too fat and decided to lose weight. Her elder sister had been told by a modelling school that one way was to induce vomiting by putting a finger down her throat. Sandra decided to do this but was disappointed that little weight loss occurred, so she accepted her existing weight as normal and ceased to worry about it. She began swimming competitively and by the age of 17 felt fit, competent, confident, and had lost 6 kg (13 lbs).

Her eighteenth year was one of tragedy. Her mother was killed in a car accident, leaving two younger children. Her older sister became a drug addict and Sandra injured herself so that she had to give up swimming. She felt she could no longer cope and deferred taking her final school exams for a year. Sandra took over the responsibilities of housekeeper and looked after her younger sisters. During this period her feeling of confidence and competency disappeared. She wrote in her diary:

I know what I should be doing. I should be going out. But meeting people is a major effort and hassle for me as I feel so uncomfortable and inept in company, especially in arranging to go to new places and meeting new people, that I end up settling for my own company. Food and eating has become such an integral part of everything. I don't want to be like this but what I eat rules my life so that every waking minute seems occupied with thoughts of food and the day passes in the measured times between when I last ate and when I'll eat again. I dream of the perfect day when I have no appetite and no thought, desire or temptation for food or to eat.

Case history: Sandra (continued)

When she was 19 she returned to complete her final exams at the local technical college, where comments about her 'emaciation' induced her to eat more. Increasing her food intake was associated with episodes of binge-eating which alarmed her. She began to induce vomiting (remembering her sister's advice) by putting her fingers down her throat. Soon she was inducing vomiting up to ten-times a day. It became increasingly difficult to dispose of the vomit. She resorted to vomiting into plastic bags and disposing of these in the garbage bin. Her father found out what she was doing and insisted that she visit a doctor, who made a diagnosis of anorexia nervosa as her weight was 39 kg (86 lbs, 6 st 2 lbs; BMI 13.8). He arranged for her to be admitted to hospital to help her gain weight and to stop her vomiting. In hospital she was co-operative and liked by the staff. A psychiatric consultation showed no major psychiatric illness. She was able to continue studying while in hospital and after discharge sat for and passed the examination. Her weight was now 46 kg (102 lbs, 7 st 4 lbs; BMI 16.3). She persisted in dieting and in self-induced vomiting and became weak. This induced her to seek re-admission to hospital. The vomiting led to a low level of potassium in her blood and tissues. She was treated with potassium supplement and an intravenous infusion.

Over the next three years during a university course she had six re-admissions to hospital for the effects of self-induced vomiting which led to a low body potassium and dehydration. These in turn caused heart-beat problems (cardiac arrhythmias) and a degree of renal failure. The admissions followed periods of increased binge-eating and vomiting which Sandra related to stress from family problems. She battled against treatment saying that her illness was 'all my fault because I will go on vomiting' and resolved each day to stop. But each day she broke her resolution when she panicked about becoming fat and when she ate food. Although she was watched by her family she managed to dispose of her vomit by hiding it in the garden or in plastic bags which she took to the university where she disposed of it. Sandra's illness became the scape-goat for the family's problems which were considerable.

Her father remarried during this time and on obtaining her degree Sandra left home. Over the next three years her weight increased slowly and is now 54 kg (119 lbs, 8 st 7 lbs; BMI 19). She no longer induces vomiting. When last contacted she said 'I look back in horror and wonder if it was some terrible nightmare.'

may cause potassium depletion and they choose foods which are low in energy but rich in potassium (such as orange juice, tomatoes, and capsicum).

The hormonal changes in anorexia nervosa

Although the decreased secretion of the hormones which are involved in menstruation are the most obvious hormonal changes accompanying anorexia nervosa (see pages 153–6), other hormonal changes occur. Laboratory studies show that the blood levels of most hormones are lowered, with the exception of cortisone, which is raised. One important change is that the function of the thyroid gland is reduced (hypothyroidism). This in turn leads to the slow heart-rate and dry skin reported by some sufferers.

When the woman's weight returns to and is maintained in the normal range, her hormone levels also return to normal. In other words they are due to low body weight and are not the cause of anorexia nervosa. They may be seen as the body's way of conserving energy, and hence of survival in face of starvation.

Psychological disturbances in anorexia nervosa (Table 20)

During severe famines, as people become emaciated and biochemical changes occur, it is common to find that their personality changes, and they tend to become apathetic, depressed, irritable, irrational, or emotionally labile, with violent swings of mood. These symptoms vary from day to day or week to week. Many victims of famine become obsessional, developing a preoccupation about food or developing abnormal taste preferences. These psychological changes are, in part, due to brain dehydration, as the brain actually becomes smaller.

As the person regains some of the weight lost during the period of starvation, these psychological changes are reversed, although the process may take some time.

Similar psychological disturbances occur in anorexia nervosa patients and disappear when the woman is re-fed and her weight increases. These findings indicate that the severe undernutrition associated with the eating disorder is the cause of the psychological changes.

Table 20. The psychological changes which may accompany anorexia nervosa

- Irritability
- Confusion
- Depressed mood (feeling hopeless, guilty, worthless)
- Insomnia
- Perfectionism
- Obsessive-compulsive behaviour, particularly about food

Many anorexia nervosa sufferers are hyperactive, always doing things and unable to relax. The hyperactivity may cause insomnia, especially early morning waking, in some sufferers.

A more unusual psychological disturbance is that anorexia nervosa (and bulimia nervosa) sufferers are more likely to shop-lift than 'normal' eaters. In a study reported from the USA in 1990, one anorexia nervosa sufferer in three either shop-lifted or stole, and many tended to harm. The reason for this psychological disturbance is unclear.

Case history: Debbie
Debbie was caught shop-lifting two children's pillow-cases and a box of chocolates. Ten days later she wrote:
For the life of me I cannot believe why I did such a stupid and criminal act. Do I put it down to another destructive coping mechanism like that of anorexia and bulimia which has been so familiar to me for the past ten years? That is what I have to believe in order to come to terms with it and at the same time learn that I need to find other methods of coping with whatever pressures I may be under. The humiliation of that day and the repercussions are just not worth it. How could I explain to the lady who caught me what I was going through and that she should know that normally I just wouldn't do something like this? I actually tried but she told me that I was just the same as all the others and that it's a shame people like me don't go to jail. The silly thing is that I had more than enough money in my purse to pay for the things I'd taken and I think that only made things worse.

Case history: Debbie (continued)
From here on, I think my body and mind relented to whatever was to happen and so as I was escorted from the shopping centre by two police officers, pushing my 21-month-old baby in her stroller, I convinced myself that people weren't staring at me and anyway this wasn't happening. Even at the police station, being questioned, finger-printed, formally charged, and a Court date given, I was oblivious to the reality of all that had happened and left the police station in a very dejected state, knowing that I had to explain all of this to my husband.

The physical disturbances (Table 21)

The physical disturbances that affect anorexia nervosa sufferers are a consequence of these biochemical and hormonal changes and the loss of body fat. To conserve energy the woman's heart-rate slows, often only beating 40 times a minute. In spite of this, if she undertakes vigorous exercise, her heart-rate increases, in a manner similar to that of 'normal' women. Her blood pressure is usually low. These two changes may lead to dizziness in some sufferers and occasionally, fainting. The woman's skin may become dry and scaly while soft, downy hair may develop on her face and body. Because she has very little fat beneath her skin, she loses her insulation. Her hands and feet feel cold and often look blue.

Some anorexia nervosa sufferers develop dental problems, particularly those who induce vomiting. The main problem is a loss of dental enamel, due to the effects of the acid vomit on the teeth. In addition dehydration, by altering the quantity and composition of the saliva increases the likelihood of dental damage. The teeth become chipped, 'moth-eaten', and may be decayed.

The lack of food and the biochemical changes lead to dilation of the intestines which gives the woman a feeling of being bloated and which may aggravate constipation. Swelling of her feet and legs (oedema) may occur, particularly following attempts to gain weight by eating more food. If the abdominal discomfort is great or the oedema noticeable, the woman may be discouraged from eating more food or may resort to taking diuretics. Oedema may also occur when she ceases to take diuretics or purgatives because of 'rebound' fluid retained in her body. She may interpret the bloating or oedema as weight gain and not fluid retention. She may then become 'panicky'

Table 21. The physical changes which may be found among women suffering from anorexia nervosa

Emaciation
Slow heart beat (and pulse)
Low blood pressure
Bloating
Constipation
Swelling of hands and feet (oedema)
Dry scaly skin
Appearance of fine facial and body hair (lanugo)
Some loss of head hair
Feeling of being cold
Absent menstruation (amenohorrhoea)
Mild anaemia

about the increase in weight and may start using dangerous methods of weight control to counter her mistaken belief that the weight gain is increased fat deposition.

Menstrual disturbances in anorexia nervosa

I haven't had my periods for the last 10 years. I have forgotten that it is normal to have periods—and not normal to be without them. Even though it seems a lot easier and convenient for them to be non-existent, I'm also aware that I'm not experiencing the emotional state of a fully developed woman because of the shut-down of my hormonal system. I find that I am feeling deprived of this privilege but the only way to regain my periods, is to do the positive thing that will remedy this situation—eat!

A major physical problem among females who have anorexia nervosa is that they fail to reach menarche, or their menstrual periods cease, often before much weight has been lost. Indeed, the absence of menstruation (amenorrhoea) is one of the features of anorexia nervosa. This can remain undetected if the woman is taking oral contraception or other hormones.

The explanation of the menstrual disturbances is rather complex, as it involves the interplay of a number of hormones (Fig. 14). The control of these hormonal relationships is situated in the area of the brain called the hypothalamus, which in turn is influenced by messages from other parts of the brain, and from outside, such as an emotional shock.

In childhood, before puberty, throughout the reproductive years, and into old age the hypothalamus secretes and releases several hormones into small blood vessels which carry them to the pituitary gland where they induce the synthesis and release of pituitary hormones, which have profound effects on the body. Because they cause the pituitary gland to release hormones, the hormones made in the hypothalamus are called releasing hormones.

The releasing hormone concerned with ovulation and menstruation is called the gonadotrophic releasing hormone or GnRH. In childhood, a small but constant amount of GnRH is released, but in the years just prior to the onset of menstruation a change occurs and GnRH begins to be released in pulsatile surges throughout the day. These pulsatile surges begin when the girl begins to grow rather rapidly in the three or four years before menarche. When her body reaches a 'critical' weight, or more accurately when the proportion of fat in her body exceeds a critical level, she menstruates for the first time, reaching menarche. Once menarche has been reached, GnRH continues to be released in a pulsatile manner throughout the reproductive years, the quantity varying from day to day. For example, during menstruation a large surge of GnRH occurs and this stimulates specialized cells in the pituitary gland to synthesize and to release follicle-stimulating hormone (or FSH). As its name implies, FSH stimulates the growth of a number of egg-containing structures (follicles) in the ovary. At puberty each ovary contains over 200 000 follicles. Each month between puberty and menopause, 10 to 20 follicles are stimulated to grow, one of them out-stripping all the others. As they develop, they synthesize the female sex hormone, oestrogen, and release it into the circulating blood. Oestrogen is taken up preferentially by the tissues of the genital organs and the breasts, particularly by the glandular lining, or endometrium, of the uterus and that of the breasts which are induced to develop, increasing in thickness. At the same time the rising amounts of oestrogen in the blood 'feedback negatively' to the hypothalamus and to the pituitary gland, leading to a slow fall in the amount of GnRH released and consequently in a fall

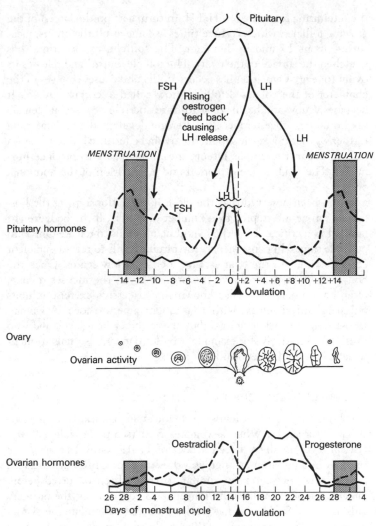

Fig. 14. The control of menstruation.

in FSH. At midcycle, that is about 16 days before the next menstrual period, a surge of oestrogen secretion occurs, causing a 'positive feedback' to the hypothalamus and to the pituitary. In response the pituitary releases both a surge of FSH and a surge of a second hormone, the luteinizing hormone or LH. LH, in turn, acts on the largest of the growing follicles, which is three times as large as all the others, measuring about 23 mm in diameter. The follicle, by this time, has stretched the surface of the ovary. The follicle 'bursts' and releases its ovum (or egg). Ovulation has occurred. LH also causes changes in the character of the collapsed follicle, now called a 'corpus luteum'. It becomes yellow and begins to synthesize and release a second female sex hormone, progesterone. Progesterone develops the endometrium further, so that it is ready should the ovum be fertilized. If fertilization fails to occur, the corpus luteum dies, and ceases to produce hormones. This leads to menstruation and a repetition of the hormonal cycle.

It has been observed that the close interrelationships of the hormones can be interrupted by a number of factors. If the body weight falls below a critical level, the hypothalamus fails to release GnRH in pulsatile surges. In consequence, the pituitary fails to release sufficient FSH to stimulate the ovaries, and menstruation ceases. Once the body weight increases above the critical level, the menses resume, often after a delay. It is also known that excessive exercise inhibits pulsatile GnRH release with consequent amenorrhoea. A woman whose weight is below normal, but above the critical level, and who exercises excessively, for example a ballet dancer, also fails to menstruate, becoming amenorrhoeic.

The effect of the hormonal changes

The hormonal changes discussed provide an explanation for the menstrual disturbances. When a woman's BMI (see p. 24) falls below a critical level usually between a BMI of 17–19, GnRH ceases to be released in a pulsatile manner, and the surges of GnRH are replaced by a steady low secretion, similar to that which occurred before puberty. Because GnRH is no longer released in surges, the pituitary fails to release FSH and LH at levels sufficient to stimulate the ovaries to secrete sufficient amounts of the female sex hormones and amenorrhoea results.

Osteoporosis

If the period of amenorrhoea lasts for longer than six months, the woman should consider taking an oral contraceptive pill or, if she prefers, the regimen of hormone replacement recommended for menopausal women. The reason for this advice is that oestrogen deprivation over a period of months leads to a loss of bone density, in other words, the bones become less strong. This may have serious consequences in later life as the woman has a greater chance of developing osteoporosis, and of having bone fractures. In her fifties and sixties the fractures most commonly occur in the bones which make up the spine (the vertebrae). In many cases the fractures cause backache and, if one or more of the vertebrae collapses, the woman becomes shorter and bent. After the age of 70, the woman has an increased risk of having a fractured hip.

The chance of these distressing events occurring is reduced considerably if a young woman's ovaries produce sufficient oestrogen and her diet contains a fair amount of calcium, so that her bones become as dense and strong as they can. The amount of oestrogen is sufficient if she menstruates regularly. She should eat at least 1 g of calcium a day, usually in the food she chooses. If she does this her bones will reach their peak density when she is about 25 years old. Provided her ovaries continue to produce oestrogen, her bones will remain at their peak density until she is 45 years old. After this time there is a slow loss of bone, which increases when she reaches the menopause.

A woman who does not menstruate regularly does not produce sufficient oestrogen to build up and to maintain the peak bone density. For this reason a young woman who has anorexia nervosa and whose periods have ceased for six months, should think about taking a hormone replacement such as the contraceptive pill until her periods return, and after that if she is sexually active and wishes for contraception. Oral contraception should not be considered substitute for the woman's own hormones as recent research suggests the benefits of oral contraception are small, even when calcium supplements are also taken. The less time women remain at low body weights the more modest the bone loss and the greater the chance of recovery to normal levels.

It is interesting that between 10 and 20 per cent of anorexia nervosa patients develop amenorrhoea before any weight loss has occurred (in fact their weight may even be increasing). Menstruation usually starts again when the woman's body weight increases to reach a BMI of 19 or more, but some women recommence menstruating at a lower body weight.

The return of menstruation

Because of the uncertainty about when ovulation and menstruation will recommence, sexually active women who do not intend to become pregnant (and babies born to women of low body weight have an increased chance of being underweight for age at birth) should not rely on lack of menstruation as protection. Some women have conceived whilst still at low body weight and having had no periods for several years. For this reason the woman or her partner should use a contraceptive method (preferably the Pill to protect her against bone loss as well as an unwanted pregnancy).

On the other hand, some women do not start menstruating again for some months, or even years, after returning to a normal body weight range. If a detailed history is taken from these women it is usually found that they have been using weight-losing methods such as excessive exercise, self-induced vomiting, and laxative abuse before weight loss or during and after weight gain. In these cases the menstrual disturbance is almost certainly associated with the weight-losing behaviour.

However, not all patients who continue to have amenorrhoea before they have lost much weight, or after refeeding, use such methods, so that some other explanation is possible. At present we do not know what it is.

Case history: Maria
Maria is the attractive youngest daughter of a family who emigrated to Australia before she was born. At the age of 14, a year after her menstrual periods started, she became aware that her family were fat, and she did not want to become fat like them. Her weight was within the desirable range at 47.5 kg (105 lbs, 7st 7 lbs; BMI 20.6) and she was teased at school as being a 'sexy Italian'. She bought some slimming tablets from the chemist, but after taking them for 5 days stopped because they 'did no good'. As her friends at school were dieting, she decided to do so too. Her plan was to eat normally for one day and starve the next day. She tended to overeat when not starving so that after two months she had gained, not lost, 4 kg (9 lbs). She heard that if she took laxatives she would lose weight, and as her mother had given laxatives to the family when they had not opened their bowels, felt she had 'permission' to use laxatives to lose weight. She also started exercising, spending 1 or 2 hours a day in exercise, telling the family she was preparing for the school sports.

Case history: Maria (continued)

Within a month of starting the exercise programme, her menstrual periods ceased, although she had only lost 2 kg (4 lbs). Maria was secretly pleased that she had no periods but was worried that people might know and wonder if she was normal. For the next five months, in spite of exercise and laxatives, her weight remained the same. In desperation to lose weight Maria refused to eat with the family as the food was 'all pasta and unhealthy'. By the age of 16, she was dieting rigidly and was abusing laxatives. Her weight began to decrease and on her 18th birthday she weighed 31 kg (68 lbs, 4 st 12 lbs; BMI 13.5). Her parents now intervened. She was admitted to hospital with a diagnosis of anorexia nervosa and started on a refeeding programme.

After three months when she was discharged from hospital her weight had increased to 49 kg (108 lbs, 7 st 10 lbs; BMI 21.3) and she had a menstrual period. At home, she continued to be afraid of becoming fat and returned to using excessive laxatives and dieted carefully to maintain a BMI of 19. She had no further menstrual periods until a year later when she found a job and a boyfriend of whom her parents approved. She ceased taking laxatives and started menstruating in spite of the fact that her weight had fallen to 42 kg (93 lbs, 6 st 9 lbs; BMI 18.3).

Marriage and children

Compared with women who do not have an eating disorder, anorexia nervosa patients after treatment are twice as likely to live alone and not to marry. If they do marry, they are twice as likely to remain childless. This may reflect the fact that only one quarter of recovered anorexics ovulate regularly. However treatment is available.

Infertility and anorexia nervosa

Although we have discussed the possibility of an unexpected pregnancy occurring during or after treatment of anorexia nervosa, studies made in Canada and our own studies, suggest that many women who have anorexia nervosa or bulimia nervosa are likely to be infertile (this is discussed in Chapter 4).

One of our Canadian colleagues examined 66 women attending an infertility clinic for the presence of an eating disorder, using a reliable psychometric test and an interview. She found that 1.5 per cent of the women had anorexia nervosa, 6 per cent had bulimia nervosa, and 9 per cent had an atypical eating disorder. This is a higher proportion than would be expected in the community. In each case the cause of the infertility was a lack of ovulation.

In our study of 14 women in whom the only reason for infertility was anovulation and who were to be treated with gonadotrophic releasing hormone (a fertility injection), we found that ten of the 14 women had a prior history of anorexia nervosa, and had had bulimia nervosa, one had an atypical eating disorder, and one woman was a compulsive exerciser. At the time we conducted the study, six of the 14 women still had an eating disorder and the compulsive exerciser was still compulsively exercising.

Women whose BMI is less than 19 should avoid being treated for infertility until their BMI exceeds 19. This is particularly important if the problem is that the woman is not ovulating. Drugs used to induce ovulation may cause excessive ovarian enlargement (the ovarian hypersensitivity syndrome), which in a number of cases leads to abdominal pain, fluid in the abdomen, a fall in blood pressure, and in about one-third of cases life-threatening blood coagulation changes. In time the ovaries usually become small again and the symptoms cease, but a few women become severely ill and some may require an operation.

The diet of anorexia nervosa patients

As has been mentioned earlier, anorexia nervosa patients are pre-occupied with food. They collect and read books and magazine articles relating to food, dieting, and body weight. Often they take over the food preparation, cooking, and serving food for the family. This allows the anorexic woman to control her food intake. She may also offer to do the cleaning up, which limits her time at the table and hides from her family the fact that she is not eating. In this way her preoccupation with food continues whilst she is praised by her family for her helpful behaviour.

Women with anorexia nervosa have read more about nutrition and food than the general public, although many of their perceptions about food are distorted and inaccurate and much of their knowledge is related to weight loss, rather than nutrition for health. Some of the false perceptions relate to the woman herself; for example, she may believe that she cannot interact with other people unless she loses weight.

Anorexia nervosa sufferers avoid eating all food types in their diet and avoid eating fat more than other foods. In a recent study made in Sydney, 17 patients who had been ill with anorexia nervosa for less than 15 months volunteered to be interviewed by a dietitian on two occasions: from these interviews typical daily food intakes were reconstructed, and the diet eaten by the women at the peak of their illness was compared with that of 'normal' women of similar age. The diet of a patient with anorexia nervosa contained one-sixth the energy, one-sixth the carbohydrate, one-third the protein, and one-tenth the fat of a normal woman's diet.

As a group these women showed wide variations in their nutrient intakes, reflecting the beliefs about and attitudes to food they held at the time. Women who resemble anorexia nervosa patients, but differ because they do not wish to change their weight or shape and pursue thinness (anorexia nervosa not for weight or shape Annws see page 34) may have diets with an even lower fat content. These women desire to 'eat healthily' usually by eliminating as much fat as they can from their diet. They read and retain the information contained on food labels and may travel long distances to obtain food brands containing the lowest fat content.

The treatment of anorexia nervosa*

It's about time I got over my anorexia, and I agree that I've wasted enough time on it. But at times I think that I hang on to my old patterns of eating behaviour, or really non-eating behaviour, as the only secure thing I can fashion from such a changing and, as I feel sometimes, topsy-turvy life. I often feel that is the only part of my life over which I can exercise any sort of control, though it ends up in the absurdity of feeling that every bit is an act of losing control.

Before any treatment is offered, the therapist must have taken a careful history to confirm that the woman has anorexia nervosa and that her body weight is not low as a consequence of experimenting with dieting, her choice of career, or her lifestyle. The doctor also makes a careful physical examination and may order some laboratory tests (Table 22).

The importance of distinguishing between women who have anorexia nervosa and women who maintain a low body weight for other reasons is shown by Zoe's story.

Zoe had always wanted to be a ballet dancer, and at the age of 15 was selected by her ballet teacher to compete for a place in a prestigious full-time ballet school. Her teacher had impressed on her the need to be thin and had weighed her once a week from the age of 12, praising her for keeping thin. Zoe said she had never had to control her weight consciously as she went to ballet classes three evenings each week, and didn't eat between school and the class. When she was weighed six months before the selection process her ballet teacher told her that she would have to lose some weight or she would not be selected. At that time her BMI was 18.5.

She started dieting and soon her weight loss was noticed by the headmistress of her school who contacted Zoe's mother fearing that Zoe was another girl who had anorexia nervosa. Her mother at once took Zoe to a doctor who arranged for her to be admitted to hospital for refeeding. Her BMI was now 16. In hospital she refused to eat, or gave her food to other patients. She adopted this strategy because she believed that if she gained weight her chance of selection to the ballet school would be jeopardized. Her resistance to refeeding confirmed to the health professionals that Zoe had anorexia nervosa. She was also considered by them to be uncooperative, untruthful, and difficult.

After three weeks in hospital she had failed to gain any weight, and after discussion was taken home by her parents. She was then referred to one of us. When we talked to Zoe, her fear of not being

Table 22. Laboratory investigations in anorexia nervosa

- full blood count and erythrocyte sedimentation rate (ESR), as sepsis may occur in the absence of fever
- blood electrolytes
- blood glucose (random sample)
- liver function tests
- renal function tests
- electrocardiogram

* See p. 188 for a summary.

selected for the ballet school became clear. We reassured her that in Australia, ballet dancers needed to have a BMI of at least 18, or they would 'not look good on stage'. Zoe accepted the reassurance and gained weight in the next five weeks, which brought her weight into the desired range.

She was selected to train at the ballet school and has maintained her weight within the range acceptable for a dancer since that time. She does not appear to be more preoccupied about food, dieting, or her weight than the other students, and is enjoying the training at which she has been very successful.

The reverse situation of that of Zoe can also occur, when the diagnosis of anorexia nervosa may be difficult as many young women who have the disorder initially deny that they have it.

Psychological management

Anorexia nervosa is a psychosomatic disorder, during which psychological and physical symptoms develop because of the self-induced starvation and other methods of inducing weight loss. The main treatment is psychological, involving cognitive behaviour therapy, supportive psychotherapy, nutritional information, and counselling about eating and potentially dangerous methods of losing weight. When appropriate, other psychological techniques, such as relaxation, interpersonal therapy, family therapy, or marital therapy may be needed. Psychological changes may be slow and early in treatment sufferers and their families may wonder if psychological treatment is effective. Over a longer time, sometimes 2 to 5 years, unhelpful and sometimes destructive attitudes about eating and body image are slowly replaced by constructive and positive thoughts and behaviours. The different types of psychological treatment are described in General management of eating disorders, Chapter 7. It is the therapist, in discussion with the patient, who suggests and decides upon the appropriate types of management at different stages of treatment.

The following was written by a patient in response to a task set by her dietitian/psychologist. Elle was asked if she would like to compare the promises her illness had made to her with what in reality had occurred:

The labyrinth
Promise: Order and satisfaction in your life. *Reality*: Disappointment and depression

Promise: Discipline and control. *Reality*: Confusion and uncertainty
Promise: Popularity and sociability. *Reality*: Isolation and loneliness
Promise: Respect and admiration. *Reality*: Pity
Promise: Perfection in all areas of life. *Reality*: Physical and mental self-destruction

Anorexia is a labyrinth of lies and destruction. No matter what options or solutions it may offer to you every choice will ultimately end in sadness and solitude. It works in the utmost deceiving and almost undetectable ways burying your true personality nearly to the point that even you may find it hard to recognise that once happy, vibrant person you were and still can be. The truth and reality I have learned, is that its power is merely an illusion. I simply had to believe I was stronger and gradually dig up those characteristics that represent me as a confident and content individual, buried beneath the lies of anorexia.

Often it's hard to believe I have it in me to fight because again and again anorexia tells me I have nothing to fight for that is worthy enough to save from destruction. But this is where I have to pay careful attention to the people around me, making a conscious effort to listen, believe and most importantly 'remember' (not dismiss) compliments and virtues they claim they saw and still see in me (despite anorexia's efforts to bury them!).

Anorexia creates its rituals through obsession and fear. The trick is to untrain these as rapidly as it trains. In the beginning it was an effort to force myself to ignore anorexia and create new habits—but if I listened to my heart, friends, and family—they always guided me whenever I questioned my actions.

You *are able* to train yourself back into reality and normality no matter how unattainable it may seem at the time.

Whenever I feel myself weakening in the fight and hear anorexia's criticisms polluting my mind, I hold onto memories of the past—how I was liked, happy, relaxed, and content, and I work on regaining these attributes. No one and certainly no disease of any kind has the power to change or destroy your memories of the past—so this is *my power* that anorexia cannot touch.

Rather than fighting the thoughts in my mind which tends to be confusing and a no win situation I have learned to fight 'Anorexia'. I question its answers, disobey its orders knowing its evil.

Destroy it before it can destroy you and win the fight—I think this is truly an opportunity to achieve something many will never even begin to understand.

In the past many treatments for anorexia nervosa have been suggested and used, such as insulin shock therapy, force-feeding, 'sleep therapy', and using medications to stimulate appetite. These should not be used. Treatment should allow patients to learn or relearn normal eating behaviour in a way that causes minimal feelings of loss of control, and panic. Drugs are seldom necessary but they may be needed in certain cases; for example, if a patient is clinically depressed she may need anti-depressants or if she has an infection she may need antibiotics. The mood of many patients improves when they are eating an adequate amount of food to ensure their bodies are no longer nutritionally deprived.

Anorexia nervosa patients are individuals. They have different problems, different needs, and are at different stages of their illness when they come for treatment—they need treatment by a person who can offer sympathetic understanding and individual treatment. This can be done by a multidisciplinary team as long as there is one consistent person in the team to whom the patient can relate and who can coordinate treatment.

Multidisciplinary teams

The varied needs of a woman suffering from anorexia nervosa frequently call for a multidisciplinary approach. The team is usually led by a psychiatrist or a clinical psychologist, but the team's dietitian has a vitally important role, as have the specialist nursing staff. The time being spent with an individual health professional depends on the patient's current needs and the relationships formed—for example, the dietitian may be the main therapist in certain cases.

The principal problem in treatment is that the patient wants to eat but is terrified that if she does so she will lose control of her eating and be unable to limit her weight gain. For this reason the hope expressed by parents, partner, or friends of an anorexia nervosa victim that 'All she has to do to get better is to eat' is unrealistic and counter-productive. The fear of losing control often extends to other aspects of the patient's life, but is particularly relevant to body weight and to food intake. For example, the fear of losing control over body weight prevents the patient from eating more than the amount she has set herself as she believes that if she eats what 'other people eat' she will put on weight rapidly. Because of this fear, patients weigh themselves daily or more often, and if they find that they have gained 1 kg (2 lbs) for no apparent reason immediately restrict the amount of food they eat or use some other method of losing weight. Even when they are emaciated they often find it safer to underestimate the amount of food they eat, rather than risk losing control over eating. As anorexia nervosa patients love food, this need to control their food intake may cause psychological turbulence. They are fearful that if they permit themselves to eat, they may be unable to stop, and that they will go on an eating binge. As many have experienced binge-eating before and after developing anorexia nervosa, the fear is real to them and it requires considerable patience by the therapist to dispel it.

Who should treat a young woman with anorexia nervosa?

The decision about who should treat a woman who has anorexia nervosa depends on the severity of the disorder, the accessibility of an experienced family doctor and a dietitian, or an eating disorders unit, and the wishes of the patient and her family.

Many young anorexia nervosa sufferers who have only recently lost weight and whose BMI is greater than 16 or who have partially relapsed following treatment in hospital, can be treated by their family doctor together with a dietitian, provided both have an interest in and experience with the eating disorder. This combination of health professionals can provide the expertise to help the majority of young women who have problems associated with strict dieting and consequent weight loss.

If however the woman does not change her eating behaviours and increase her weight, more specialized help is indicated. This may involve her attending a specialized eating disorder unit as an outpatient, a day-patient, or requiring treatment in hospital.

For many young women, attendance at a specialized Eating Disorder Unit as a day-patient from the start of treatment is possible. Day-patient treatment allows the woman to live at home whilst attending each day the specialized eating disorder unit where she receives help to make the changes needed for her recovery. Her daily attendance at the eating disorder unit gives her access to a team of supportive and experienced people who can help her cope with the range of problems she experiences. One disadvantage of this programme is that it does not allow the young woman to attend her place of education, training, or work.

Table 23. Indications for admission to hospital

• very low body weight with life-threatening physiological changes (see page 152)

• serious cardiac and electrolyte disturbances

• need to separate the patient from family problems

• possible risk of suicide

• lack of response to out-patient treatment

As many anorexia nervosa patients are high achievers, their withdrawal from their place of study or work may decrease their self-esteem. This can be overcome if the patient is fit enough to be treated as an out-patient.

The advantages of being treated by an experienced family doctor and a dietitian, or attending an eating disorder unit as an out-patient or as a day-patient are as follows. First, the woman can increase her weight at her own speed so that she feels safe and in control. Second, she has to take responsibility for her eating behaviour and, with the support of her health professionals, can relearn eating patterns which are appropriate to her lifestyle.

If hospital admission is required (Table 23) or chosen, the woman, unless she is desperately ill, is first given the opportunity to be responsible for her own weight gain, with the support of the dietitian and the nursing team.

The objectives of treating anorexia nervosa

The objectives of treating anorexia nervosa are shown in Table 24, but require some further clarification.

1. *To help the patient increase her weight so that it is within the normal range.* The choice of where her weight should lie, within the normal BMI range, is a balance between the weight a woman is likely to accept (usually it is the range of a BMI of 19 to 20) and the weight which is likely to be associated with a successful outcome (that is a BMI of 20 to 25). Although it is a bit on the thin side of the normal range, the reason for choosing a BMI of 19 to 20 (which is about 90 per cent of Average Body Weight) is that in this weight range most

Table 24. The aims of treatment of anorexia nervosa

- to help the sufferer increase her weight by refeeding so that it lies between a BMI of 19 and 25
- to educate her about nutrition and normal eating behaviour and to correct erroneous beliefs about food (e.g. 'good' and 'bad' foods)
- to help her feel that she has control over her eating behaviour
- to establish normal eating behaviour and to desist from using dangerous methods of weight control
- to explain the physical symptoms of anorexia nervosa, and why and how they arise
- to deal with any associated problems, such as relationship or family problems

physiological functions, such as temperature control, menstruation, growth, and development will have returned or will soon return to normal. The weight level is also realistic as it helps the patient avoid feeling anxious about becoming fat. At this weight a young adolescent woman may be able to commence growing again and reach her expected height and development.

2. *To correct the sufferer's views about food.* We have mentioned that patients who have anorexia nervosa read a great deal about food from diet books and magazines, and in consequence tend to have more knowledge about food than the average person. However many of their opinions of food and eating are erroneous and, unless corrected, will perpetuate their eating disorder. They are also often rigid and opinionated in their beliefs. For these reasons, an important part of treatment is for the sufferer to receive educational sessions (preferably in a group setting) from a dietitian so that their distorted opinions about food, dieting, and eating behaviour are corrected.

3. *To help the sufferer feel that she has control over her abnormal eating behaviour*, so that she no longer persists with her 'relentless pursuit of excessive thinness', to quote Hilda Bruch, who was a pioneer in treating anorexia nervosa. Correcting the disordered thoughts, attitudes and feelings about body image that are thought to be central to the development and maintenance of anorexia nervosa is essential.

4. *To persuade the patient to adopt normal eating behaviour*, and to avoid starving herself, if she has restrictive anorexia nervosa. If she is a binger and purger the objective is to help her to stop using these

potentially dangerous behaviours. If she is a compulsive exerciser, this behaviour also needs to be tackled.

5. *To explain to the sufferer why she has developed the physical changes, that they are a consequence of starvation and weight-losing behaviours, and to help her correct them.*

6. *To help the sufferer deal with any associated problems which may be present or may arise during treatment.* These problems, if not addressed, may prevent recovery.

Increasing body weight

Although anorexia nervosa is a psychosomatic problem, the first priority in treatment must be to achieve weight gain, as most patients do not respond to psychological treatment at low body weight or when failing to gain weight. It is important for the patient to realize that the long-term aim is for her to learn to increase her weight and to maintain it within the normal desirable range for her age and height. This does not mean that she has to control her weight to within 0.5 kg (1 lb) on a day-to-day basis. In fact, weighing more than once a week is meaningless (unless the woman is in hospital receiving treatment) as it is normal for the weight to vary by more than 1 kg (2 lbs) over a period of days. Although a weight corresponding to a BMI of 19 is set as a target weight, this is the minimum weight for normal physiological function such as the return of menstruation. At this weight, the patient is still on the thin side of normal and as many women look better at a higher weight she may be encouraged to attempt this. There are certain exceptions; for example, if the woman is a fashion model or a ballet dancer she may not accept a weight corresponding to a BMI over 19 as desirable, and she and her therapist have to agree that a lower weight is appropriate in her case. They may also have to agree that she is likely to remain preoccupied with her weight and to limit her food intake, so that she may retain the body shape expected of her profession. A complete recovery from anorexia nervosa is associated with achieving a body weight in the normal range of BMI.

Refeeding

As mentioned earlier, refeeding is the main way in which the sufferer is helped to gain weight. During the refeeding programme, she has regular sessions with her therapist, is provided with nutritional information by her dietitian, learns to eat normally, and is helped to cope with her everyday problems, particularly if she has had anorexia nervosa for some time.

Whether she is treated as an out-patient or is admitted to hospital, she is first given the opportunity to be responsible for her own weight gain with the help of the supporting health professionals. During this time she may be ambulant, doing supervised, very low intensity exercise and attending discussion and educational sessions with other sufferers to help her gain insight into her eating disorder and any other problems. She is encouraged to pursue interests such as relaxation techniques, craft, and painting. If she is of school age, she can continue with her school curriculum with home or hospital-based programmes developed with the help of her teachers.

During refeeding she is alerted to the possibility of a rapid weight gain which occurs when refeeding begins. It results from the expansion of fluid in the tissues between the body cells (the extracellular compartment) and an increase in the body's glycogen-water pool (see page 261). This may cause great anxiety and the woman needs to be assured that the weight gain, which is due to rehydration, will resolve spontaneously if she continues to adhere to the refeeding programme.

In hospital the patient may be weighed each day at the same time of day on the same scales, but some believe that, because minor daily changes in weight occur, it is preferable to weigh the patient two or three times a week, not daily. Weighing has to be done carefully and the nurse must make sure that the patient does not cheat, for example, by drinking a litre or more of water just before being weighed or by putting weights in her pockets (Table 26). Occasional weighing at unpredictable times is used to check if the patient is cheating.

During the refeeding programme, the woman is expected to eat a varied diet, balanced in macronutrients and in micronutrients with the inclusion of 'feared' high-energy foods in moderation. The aim is for a weight increase of 1.0–1.5 kg (2–3 lbs) a week if she is in hospital and 0.3–0.5 (0.5–1 lb) a week if she is an outpatient.

In the early stages of refeeding, this weight increase can be achieved with a smaller amount of 'normal' food providing 6700–7700 kJ (1600–1800 kcals) a day, depending on the patient's nutritional intake prior to her admission. Once the woman can eat this quantity of food without purging or over-exercising, and her weight has stabilized, an increase in food intake will be necessary. This should be discussed between the patient and her dietitian.

Table 25. Cheating with food intake as told by patients

1. Hide food in table napkin or tissue
2. Leave the crust of toast or bread on the plate, discarding the rest
3. Dispose of food into vases, stuffed toys, cupboards, or out of the window
4. Keep food in the mouth and discard it when cleaning the teeth
5. Surreptitiously feed the family dog under the table
6. Keep high energy food under long fingernails and wash hands after eating.

If she feels that the amount of food is too large and too bulky—usually containing more than 12 600 kJ (3000 kcals)—then high-energy drinks or food supplements may be used. Some women need to increase their food intake to 12 600–14 500 kJ (3000–5000 kcals) a day to reach the target weight. Once this has been reached a menu providing a maintenance intake of 10 000–11 000 kJ (2400–2600 kcals) a day is constructed.

During the early part of the programme the woman, whether she is an in-patient, a day-patient, or an out-patient needs to be medically monitored to prevent potentially dangerous consequences which may occur during refeeding. If refeeding takes place too quickly the 'refeeding syndrome' may occur, during which, among other biochemical changes, much of the phosphorus in the blood is taken into the body cells leading to a low level of blood phosphate (hypophosphataemia). Death may occur unless phosphorus supplements are given. The diet is also devised to contain sufficient carbohydrate to avoid the problem of a possible metabolic ketosis.

As the programme progresses, greater amounts of food are offered and expected to be eaten so that a slow but steady weight gain is achieved.

Some women may be encouraged to recover more quickly if the woman and her therapist or dietitian agree that she may remain at the same increased weight for a week or two before another increase is expected.

Most anorexia nervosa sufferers respond to the lenient approach to treatment. If the patient refuses to be refed, an ethical problem arises about whether she should be forcibly refed against her wishes,

Table 26. Cheating to apparently increase weight as told by patients

1. Drinking large amounts of water the night before being weighed

2. Avoid emptying bladder before being weighed

3. Drinking bath or shower water

4. Binge-eating the night before

5. Wear heavy jewellery or heavy clothing (such as ski braces)

6. Sew weights into clothes or insert the weight into her bra before being weighed

or no refeeding undertaken, in which case she may die. This issue is under debate but no resolutions have been reached.

If the woman does not respond, a more structured programme should be implemented. In extreme cases the woman may have to be observed continually or kept in somewhat extreme isolation in a single-bedded room and have to stay in bed until the 'target weight' is reached by refeeding. This strategy is necessary because many patients try to find methods to avoid eating or to get rid of food by inducing vomiting or abusing laxatives (see Table 25).

If she eats the amount of food expected and conforms to treatment by avoiding weight-losing strategies, and starts gaining weight, she is offered a 'reward' or a 'privilege'. For example, she may be allowed to get up and have a shower, or to watch television. On the other hand, if she fails to put on weight she knows that privileges may be taken away and she may be ordered to go back to bed and stay there.

Although this appears to be a very strict programme, women who are at very low body-weight frequently are unable to think clearly and the fear of gaining weight is overpowering (see also page 150). Some women who have experienced refeeding will ask to go on a bed-rest programme, as will some women who are finding eating and weight gain difficult to achieve. These women see this strict programme as helpful and supportive, rather than punitive. The negative aspects reported by patients are boredom and isolation.

Naso-gastric feeding is another method of refeeding. This involves passing a thin, flexible tube into the stomach by way of the nose and oesophagus and through which measured amounts of liquid food can be given 3 or 4 times each day. The tube must be introduced by an experienced person and the patient must be carefully monitored in a medical setting throughout the refeeding period. This method is not without complications, the patient may try to remove or destroy the tube, retain too much fluid and if feeding is too rapid the 'refeeding syndrome' can occur. The patient's fluid, food, weight, and electrolytes in the blood are monitored to prevent feeding that is too rapid and that may result in cardiac arrest.

Some patients who accept they have a problem but feel unable to eat view naso-gastric feeding very positively. They may express relief that the responsibility for eating has been taken away from them. As they gain weight the intensity of their fears of eating decrease and they are able to start to eat again. This method of refeeding is being used more frequently as it means patients spend less time at low body weights and the health costs are reduced.

Some women are unable to recognise they are ill and may refuse treatment. At very low weight a woman may not be able to make an informed decision about her treatment. Anorexia nervosa patients can be very convincing in their arguments, particularly those involving weight gain, they will agree to anything that will delay weight gain and disagree with any suggestions that involve immediate treatment. They may even choose death over a life of constant vigilance against weight gain (see case study Cassandra page 37). These attitudes change as weight is gained and patients respond to adequate nutrition. When parents and doctors consider a patient is sufficiently impaired and unable to make an informed decision about accepting treatment naso-gastric feeding may be necessary.

There are both advantages and disadvantages, and advocates for and against naso-gastric feeding. The patient spends less time at low body weights; her bone loss is less and she has less time to learn and practise new weight losing behaviours and acquire additional distorted attitudes to food and eating. Tube feeding is used to help women restore their nutrition and commence putting on weight. Once part of the weight has been gained and the woman's attitudes to eating are less rigid she can start to eat and learn 'normal eating'. When patients are no longer at very low body weights they can slowly begin to participate effectively in psychological treatments, they can interact with their friends and family and return to school or work earlier than if they had not been tube fed. Treatment for anorexia nervosa is expensive; a shorter length of stay in hospital is a factor for some families and health deliverers must take this into consideration.

In addition to the 'risks' of tube feeding cited earlier in this section naso-gastric feeding does not help a woman take responsibility for her own eating and she still has to learn 'normal eating'. It is hard to compare the different types of refeeding as naso-gastric feeding is only used for severe cases of anorexia nervosa in most hospitals.

Helping the patient gain confidence

This part of the treatment is designed to help the women gain confidence. With her therapist's support and encouragement she learns how much she needs to eat to control her weight at an appropriate level. She has to be made aware that she will not be rewarded for gaining weight rapidly, as this may merely indicate that she is binge-eating.

The therapist also has the responsibility of helping the patient to adjust to the other problems (such as relationship problems) which may have arisen because of the patient's fear of losing control.

The therapist's function is to explore these problems with the patient, so that he or she gains the patient's trust, and to encourage her motivation to return to 'normal' eating. She must also give the patient the confidence to continue with treatment and must help her to maintain her body weight within the normal range.

As the therapist becomes aware of the patient's fear of losing control and her resistance to changing her eating behaviour, it may become apparent that treatment will have to be delayed until the patient is 'ready to get better', even though this means that a few patients will become severely ill and have to be rescued from impending death by urgent admission to hospital. Other patients who require admission include those who are severely ill when first seen, those who fail to make progress as an out-patient, those who persist in continuing with their weight-losing behaviour, and those who are incapable of responding to treatment as a result of the physical and mental consequences of the very low body weight. In other cases the patient's doctor may feel she should be admitted to hospital, or she herself may prefer to be treated in hospital.

During the time that she gains weight, the patient often feels 'full' and her stomach may bulge. She needs to be told that this will happen, and needs to be reassured that the abdominal swelling will not remain. Unless this is done, she may feel that she is losing control. These are temporary symptoms which the patient has to suffer to achieve her goal. The abdominal swelling is due to distension of the intestines, and, once intestinal function becomes normal, the abdomen becomes flat, whilst fat is deposited on her limbs and body. During refeeding the patient should avoid buying tight-fitting clothes, such as jeans, because within two or three weeks after her desirable weight has been achieved and the distension has subsided they will be too big. The appearance of a 'bulging stomach' is usually more marked among patients who are refed in hospital and who are not permitted to exercise, than among patients who are allowed to undertake supervised low intensity exercise.

When a reasonable amount of weight gain each week has been obtained, it will be found that the amount tapers off as the 'target' body weight range is approached. At this stage women who are patients in hospital should remain in hospital for two or three weeks after their weight is in the desirable weight range to make sure that the weight is maintained, and that they gain confidence that they can maintain their weight in the desired weight range, and can learn how much to eat.

The patient needs reassurance that her weight gain is not predominantly due to an increase in body fat. In fact during this period the body selectively gains protein, increasing the woman's lean body mass rather than her adiposity.

After achieving a body weight in the middle or upper part of her target range, the woman's diet is modified to contain slightly more energy than would be considered necessary to maintain a weight in the normal weight range, for about a month. This strategy prevents a sudden drop in body weight to below the desired weight range when refeeding stops.

Some women require higher than expected energy intakes for some weeks, or even months, if they are to maintain the desired body weight. The reason for this energy wasting in women during and after refeeding is not known.

Establishing normal eating behaviour

As most anorexia nervosa patients restrict the number of different foods they eat, the second aim of treatment is for the patient to learn to choose from a wide range of foods. This wide choice provides her body with the many nutrients it needs. She is helped to stop seeing foods as 'good' (that is, with a low energy content and low or no fat) or 'bad' (with a high energy and fat content), and learns to eat a wide variety of foods in sensible amounts (see Table 31 on page 221). Eating sensibly includes learning to eat in front of people, at different venues and in social situations, and to be comfortable about this. For example, if someone who has had anorexia nervosa goes to a social function, such as a wedding or a Chinese banquet, she may eat far more than her body requires that day and has to learn to accept that this is normal. She also has to conquer her preoccupation with food and her urge to weigh every item of food she eats and to calculate its kilojoule (calorie) content. Many patients have no idea of how much they can eat without weight gain and have trouble recognizing cues for hunger and satiation. During treatment they learn to recognize these cues and are taught the elements of dietetics. Many patients who have an eating disorder do not know what 'normal' eating is. To help them to be aware of normal eating, we have listed some of the criteria in Table 32 and 33 on pages 222–3.

These matters are explored and discussed during the educational sessions which take place concurrently with the refeeding programme. They may be discussed when the woman and her therapist meet or in group sessions led by the dietitian or one of the skilled members of the nursing staff. Many eating disorder experts believe that this 'psycho-education' is most effective if conducted with a group of patients.

Ceasing weight-losing behaviours

A major concern is to change the potentially dangerous weight-losing behaviours resorted to by many women who have anorexia nervosa. Many patients respond to information about the short- and long-term effects of vomiting and abuse of purgatives, diuretics, and slimming tablets, and are willing, at least initially, to reduce the frequency of these behaviours. They find reassurance on learning what effects to expect when they stop vomiting and using laxatives, for example, that they may undergo a temporary weight gain as they become rehydrated, and that constipation may persist for some time, as well as abdominal fullness and cramps. As the patients are preoccupied with their body weight and abdominal fullness, these are the very symptoms which make them anxious and may make them return to vomiting and laxatives unless they know that these symptoms are to be expected.

Women who have anorexia nervosa may be manipulative and untruthful when they are questioned about their food intake and their methods of losing weight. The therapist may have to confront the patient before treatment is started, to establish, as far as possible, whether she is prepared to agree to try and eat more food. Truthful common-sense confrontation is also required during treatment if the patient is discovered cheating. For example, she may appear to take all the food offered and then dispose of most of it surreptitiously down the sink, or place weights in the pockets of her clothing when she knows that she is to be weighed. She may exercise frenetically in her room or in the shower or bathroom, where she knows that she can do it secretly. She may also secretly resort to self-induced vomiting or abuse laxatives when she decides that she has reached a certain weight and does not want to gain more, as she is fearful that she is losing control of her eating.

Explaining the physical symptoms

Some patients are content that they no longer menstruate, but if they are in their late-teens or twenties they may need reassurance that menstruation will return if they maintain their higher weight, stop extreme methods of weight control, exercising excessively, and abusing laxatives, enemas and diuretics, although the return of menstruation may be delayed for several months. As the patient gains weight she may want her menstrual periods to start again as she sees this as a demonstration that she is getting better. Other women require discussion and reassurance that their dry skin, broken hair, and lanugo hair will disappear as their nutrition improves.

The place of exercise during treatment

Studies have shown that women who have anorexia nervosa gain weight faster if their activity is limited during treatment. For this reason, it would appear sensible to limit a woman's activity to reduce the time she remains at low body weight.

There are other factors, however, to be considered. These include the quality of the patient's life, how she feels and looks, and the need for her to learn or relearn what is 'normal activity' and what is 'sensible activity'. Treatment is also directed to encourage the weight gain to be partly lean (muscle) body weight as well as the increased deposition of body fat.

In the general community, exercise is encouraged so that conditions such as obesity are avoided, the chance of having a heart attack is reduced, and the mobility of joints is maintained. Most people say that they feel better about themselves and their body if they exercise regularly. Also, women who are trying to gain weight find that regular exercise reduces the size of the abdomen by redistributing fat and increasing intestinal tone.

Graduated, controlled exercise during the refeeding period of an anorexia nervosa sufferer increases the recovery of lean body mass by increasing the muscle mass. As some women who have anorexia nervosa immediately reduce their food intake once they have reached their target weight range and in consequence lose some of the fat they had deposited during refeeding, the greater the proportion of weight gained as lean body mass, the better the long-term outcome may be. This avoids a woman being discouraged by observing her temporary loss of body weight.

As we noted earlier in this chapter, many anorexia nervosa patients exercise excessively and many others appear to be continually active or hyperactive. If these women are denied the opportunity to exercise, the result may be agitation and the woman may continue exercising in secret. In most cases the woman does not know how much exercise she is doing and cannot equate her secret exercise with what is appropriate for her after refeeding.

It seems sensible for an anorexia nervosa patient, if she so wishes, to embark on a graduated exercise programme whilst under treatment so that she may learn and accept a sensible exercise programme which is appropriate for her and which aims to achieve the levels of exercise she is likely to do after leaving hospital. This allows the woman to learn what exercise is safe and 'normal'. However, if the woman is not gaining weight whilst being re-fed, the amount of exercise she does must be reduced or may have to stop.

Exercise disorder

A sensible exercise programme which the woman does during refeeding and during the maintenance of her body weight in the target weight range may prevent her from replacing the eating disorder with an exercise disorder. In this, the pursuit of thinness and a preoccupation with body weight, shape, and food intake is replaced by a preoccupation with exercise, body building, and body shape, which can be just as disabling as the previous eating disorder.

Case history: Dorothy
There's no question about it, it has to be done. It's like I can't see beyond the actual obsession. I can't do anything to distract myself. I wouldn't know what to do till I'd done it. I just hurry and get it over—done with as fast as possible so I can relax. It's like a duty I have to perform before I can continue with life. The stairs are the worst—I only do it at night, although the thought pops into my head every time I have to walk up or down them. It is at night when everyone is home, so I have to pick my time and walk softly. I feel everyone else is controlling when I can do it, trying to stop me. Just leave me alone and let me finish. I have to get it done! I can't live, I don't know how to live without them. If I don't do it I will be a self-indulgent, fat, lazy slob. When I'm tired, my thoughts are fuzzy, so I can't figure them; when I'm alert I have enough energy to run across the Nullabor. Let me do them, get it over and done with, put it behind me, let it be over for another night. Quickly, quickly, faster and faster. Sometimes I feel so ashamed of myself for doing this—I just close my eyes or focus on how good it will be when it's all over. It's so lovely. My awareness is heightened, I can hear everything and feel everything and gosh, it hurts. Stop it, time out, defocus on what's around and just feel the ache in my legs. Just let me keep going, go and have your shower so I can do it knowing no one will interrupt me. I hate interruptions. It makes me lose count. It's cool when everyone is out or in bed—I can just go hellfire, another priority completed for the day. I'm so angry. Faster, faster, harder, harder, block everything but just keep counting. It's so insidious, like this urgent, desperate, persistent itch going on in my head, slowly becoming a roar so loud that reality is blocked out. Nobody listens, nobody hears, nobody changes. Everything is so bloody frustrating I can't ever scream out my anger because society reads it as a sign of needing help or having totally lost the plot. So what was simple frustration is now multiple compounded frustration and my head is paralysed, despite wanting to be bashed against a brick wall.

Relapses

In the first year after treatment, 20–30 per cent of anorexia nervosa patients who have apparently recovered, again lose weight and relapse into the one or more of the behaviours described on pages 171 and 172. If the woman can maintain her body weight in the normal range for a year, there is less likelihood of relapse, although it may still occur.

Dealing with associated problems

Some patients say that when they are in control of their food intake and their body weight, they feel in control of their lives. For example, when preparing for an examination the patient may feel it would be 'good' to put on weight but resists this because if she starts to lose control of her eating behaviour she fears she will lose control of her self-discipline, will not study, and will fail the examination. Her control of her eating behaviour may continue for other reasons. It may become part of a reward-punishment system. She may argue: 'If I eat one extra thing, something dreadful will happen to me'. It may be used to manipulate parents or her husband, to gain attention, or as an excuse if she does not perform as well as they expect: 'If I am thin, people know there is something wrong and do not expect as much.'

On the other hand, some anorexia nervosa sufferers have problems which upset them and which affect their behaviour. For example, the preoccupation with weight control and with food may be used to prevent the patient thinking about her other problems. The eating disorder may also permit the woman to escape from having to make decisions and from participating in events which she fears.

Patients of ours have told us that 'people do not expect as much of you when you look sick'; and 'people treat you more gently if you have an eating disorder'; or 'it keeps my parents talking to each other'; or 'my husband will leave me if I get better'. These last two comments show that the family may be involved in producing or maintaining the eating disorder.

Although most anorexia nervosa patients have a supportive, sharing, communicating family, some form a part of a 'dysfunctional' family. These families tend to have rigid, unbending attitudes and values, or are over-protective of their children, the parents being unable to allow their children to be independent, or the family is chaotic and disorganized. These families seem to be unable to resolve problems which arise within the family, and may need a 'sick' member to enable the other family members to communicate with each other, or to take sides in parental quarrels. In these situations, family therapy may be needed if the woman is to recover.

Some older anorexia nervosa patients may feel that they cannot recover from their eating disorder whilst in their current relationship. The situation is more likely to arise if the woman married after the onset of anorexia nervosa. At that time, her husband had been attracted by a thin, fragile, dependent woman who had a problem. He may have sought a woman whom he could care for and derived much satisfaction from looking after her. If she now recovers and becomes less dependent, he may feel uncomfortable and may feel that his enjoyable role has diminished. This can lead to family problems which may need professional help to be resolved, or the couple may separate or divorce.

If family problems are revealed during talks with the sufferer, she may be helped if she talks with a therapist who has expertise in relationship and marital problems, or in family therapy. Indeed in some cases this help is essential if the eating disorder is to be resolved.

If the problem is one of adjustment to adolescence, a problem relating to sexuality, or a gynaecological problem, the woman may welcome the opportunity to talk with an appropriate expert who is chosen because of his empathy and ability to communicate well.

The parents of young women who have anorexia nervosa may equally need support. Support groups for parents can provide information and reassurance and also enable the parents to gain insight into their daughter's eating disorder.

Some women who have anorexia nervosa are helped considerably after they have been re-fed and helped to overcome their immediate problems, by joining a *self-help group* composed of anorexia nervosa sufferers and those who have almost or completely recovered from the disorder. An alternative is to join in *small-group therapy*, in which a health professional acts as a facilitator for a group of sufferers, who discuss their problems and the ways they are being helped to overcome them. Both groups are often successful if the group is made up of people with similar needs, for example, people of similar ages or people who are employed, or undertaking tertiary education, or who are married or single, or who have children.

These problems and strategies for their relief, discussed in this section, may equally apply if the woman has bulimia nervosa, the binge-eating disorder, or an eating disorder not otherwise specified.

Medications

Medications play an insignificant part in the management of anorexia nervosa. In most studies which have used antidepressants as part of the treatment, they have been prescribed because some women who have anorexia nervosa also have symptoms suggesting depression. Usually, these symptoms, which are not sufficient for a diagnosis of clinical depression, disappear as the woman gains weight and recovers. However some anorexia nervosa patients also have a moderate or even severe depressive illness, although the proportion is no higher than that among women who do not have an eating disorder. Unless the woman is severely depressed, the use of antidepressants has proved to be of little benefit, as people who are emaciated respond less well to the medications. If an antidepressive drug is needed, one of the selective serotonin reuptake inhibitors (SSRIs), such as fluoxetine or paroxetine is preferred. These drugs are very effective for women who are depressed and who suffer from obsessive-compulsive disorder (OCD) but the results from recent studies of their use in the treatment of women suffering with anorexia nervosa have been disappointing. It is possible there may be a role for these drugs in the subsequent phase of treatment, during weight maintenance, particularly if a woman is distressed by her mood at this time.

Anorexia nervosa patients are also more likely than people of normal weight to develop unpleasant side-effects which are occasionally life-threatening, for example, cardiac arrhythmias.

The prevention of relapses

Women who have required treatment in hospital are more vulnerable to relapse than those who have been less ill and have been treated as out-patients. During the recovery period the woman should have continuing contact with her dietitian and the therapist at varying intervals. In addition, the woman should know that she can contact her dietitian or her therapist at any time.

A second group of patients who may need continuing help are those who have apparently recovered from anorexia nervosa, but are worried that a relapse is about to occur. It is important for these women to know that they can quickly obtain help from a therapist whom they trust and with whom they feel comfortable.

Some women are unable to achieve the desired body weight even after treatment. Their body weight stabilizes at a weight well below the normal range. These women cannot be considered 'cured' as they continue to be preoccupied with thoughts about weight and food, continue a rigid lifestyle to maintain their restricting behaviour, and tend to avoid challenges to this way of life. In other words their eating disorder continues to interfere with their daily living. They are particularly likely to have a relapse during which their weight decreases and they become ill.

Other women, whose weight has returned to the normal range, but who continue to be preoccupied, to some extent, with thoughts of weight and food, may relapse if they have a life stress or some other challenge, such as an impending examination, a change of job, illness, marriage, or divorce. Some women with anorexia nervosa replace their abnormal eating behaviour with an exercise disorder or alcohol dependence, during which they may relapse into a further episode of anorexia nervosa.

As well as being able to contact their therapist easily and quickly, in many cases the relapse can be prevented if the woman follows these guidelines.

- She is aware that it is preferable for her to allow her body weight to increase a little after she has achieved the target recommended during refeeding. This permits her body to correct the ratio of lean (mostly muscle) tissue to fat tissue so that its composition is normal.
- Tries to avoid any further weight loss for any reason. For example, if she has a period of illness when she loses weight she should try to regain that weight (even if it is only a kilogram) as quickly as possible.
- Avoids situations which keep her thinking about food, her body shape, or weight. For this reason she should avoid working in a job involving food preparation or serving, for example, working as a waitress or in a restaurant or take-away food shop.
- Avoids changing her routine too much.
- Avoids long holidays or trips overseas. In an unfamiliar environment, with the loss of routine, frequent new experiences, and different foods, she may feel that she has lost control and reverts to

restricting her food intake or binge-eating and using dangerous compensatory methods of weight control.

Kara, a 22-year-old ex-patient of ours, returned from overseas and entered the Eating Disorders Unit for refeeding. Her story is an example of what may happen if a woman who is recovering from anorexia nervosa goes overseas too early. She wrote:

Case history: Kara

I had been looking forward to the trip for months, but when I arrived at the airport the reality of going finally hit me . . . and I found myself asking 'What am I doing?' I didn't know what to expect and it was the first time I'd left home and been so far away from my parents. Plus—my eating wasn't all that stable, although I tried to ignore that fact.

In the plane I was already 'cutting back', as I wasn't flexible enough to cope with the type of meals that were served, and as we changed time zones a few times, it seemed like I was faced with a roast dinner when it theoretically should have been about 3 o'clock in the morning! As I was settling into a new life, I was always looking in the shops for the types of food I was used to eating at home and felt safe with. I became aware that I was trying to take Australia with me, and found it difficult to accept a different culture and cuisine, due to the rigidity of my habitual daily intake.

As it was winter, we ate a lot of heavy foods, such as potatoes with creamy sauces, fatty meats, and greasy vegetables. This, as well as the custom of eating the main meal in the middle of the day, was guilty and anxiety-producing for me, as I kept thinking of my meal sitting there in my stomach the whole afternoon. To combat this, I often went for a bike ride or to the local swimming pool. I tried to occupy myself as much as possible with study, writing letters, and going out, so that I wouldn't be reminded that I was hungry or have an excuse to eat. I was also doing exercises every night in my room—an obsession which had started many months ago at home.

As a result of excessive exercise and eating as little as I could get away with, I kept losing weight. I also began isolating myself in my room, and feeling very lonely and depressed. I kept longing for the security of home, and became increasingly withdrawn and secretive, bottling up my emotions inside and believing no one could possibly understand.

By this stage I was so caught up in my own thoughts that I could see no other way but down. It was like my eating disorder was ruling me again, and I was made aware of how powerful it is.

Case history: Kara (continued)

Finally, after much crying and frantic deliberation, I decided the best thing for me to do would be to come home and get proper treatment in hospital. I had lost about 5 kg in 7 weeks, having already been underweight when I left home.

When I look back on it now, I realize how important it is to be honest with yourself when planning big changes in your life. I would not recommend that anyone who has or has had an eating disorder go overseas unless (she) is completely recovered, and has the strength to recognize her 'triggers' and instigate appropriate coping strategies. Adapting to a new situation and life-style without the 'policemen'— that is, family, friends, and doctors—can be stressful. The easiest and most natural thing to do is to resort to old coping mechanisms and behaviours, which can ultimately be destructive. The prospect of an overseas trip is of course very exciting and challenging, but you can't fit your eating disorder in your suitcase too.

The outcome of anorexia nervosa

The aims of treatment are: first, to help the woman achieve a weight within the normal body weight range, that is, a BMI of 19 or more; second, to help her to eat normally for her age and lifestyle; third, to enable her to avoid extreme methods of weight control; fourth, to enable her to gain insight so that she no longer needs her eating disorder to help her cope with problems of her daily life; fifth, to help her to improve her body image and body concept so that it no longer depends on her body weight.

Between 50 and 75 per cent of anorexia nervosa patients achieve these aims completely or partially after treatment lasting six months to six years. In other words 40–50 per cent of sufferers from anorexia nervosa will recover completely, and 30–40 per cent recover sufficiently to lead a normal life, although they may continue to have thoughts or behaviours that are associated with an eating disorder.

Recovery is more likely if she is younger, is not at very low weight, if it is the first time she has received treatment, treatment is started early, if the woman's family is supportive, if there is no conflict between family members, and if the woman was a 'dieter' rather than a 'vomiter and purger'. Unfavourable factors are a profound loss of weight, and if anorexia nervosa is associated with bulimia nervosa.

Many women who have apparently recovered may continue to need support in the following years and should know that they can obtain counselling and psychotherapy should they feel they need it.

Kylie's story typifies the problem. In the previous three years she had had four admissions to hospital for refeeding. Each admission had lasted for at least two months. After being discharged from hospital for the fourth time she wrote to the doctor:

I know that I still look too thin, but I just don't seem able to regain the weight I lost in the last four months. It may be because I left home then. I was very worried about how I'd cope when I started living away from home again, and tried to be strict with myself about 'cutting back' on food. I don't think I did 'cut back', but suppose I'm a lot more active now at work than I was when I was at home leading a life of (enforced) leisure. However, I find it almost impossible to let myself eat more. As you may remember, my problem has always been an 'eating-food' one, rather than a concern with weight. Basically I still think the same way as I have for a long time, and I don't suppose this will ever change now.

Anorexia now seems to be becoming increasingly common, and receiving a lot of publicity. I don't know whether the publicity is all for the good—I have the feeling it may be becoming almost 'fashionable' among young girls, without their realising its long-term consequences. If I could but turn the clock back about twelve years; wishful thinking!

A year later, Kylie wrote again:

Considering everything, I've been keeping quite well. I've maintained my weight since I left the Clinic (over a year ago now!) though I haven't put any more on. I'm still not over-confident about how I would cope on my own, i.e. if I was preparing and responsible for all my own food. So many of the old attitudes are still lying dormant and I have to be ever vigilant that they don't exert too much influence. All in all it's still not terribly easy, though I must admit that I do think less and less about being an 'anorexic'.

The remaining 15–25 per cent of anorexia nervosa patients continue to suffer from anorexia nervosa, requiring intermittent therapy over many years. The last two groups of patients require the support of, and to be counselled by, a therapist at intervals for several years after refeeding, because life and developmental stresses may precipitate a recurrence. Refeeding, re-education of eating habits, and explanation of physical symptoms are only initial goals in the treatment of anorexia nervosa.

Helping the woman to understanding what is happening and to give her reassurance about these matters and her beliefs about eating is equally important. Although this information is given during the refeeding period, most patients have more insight and understanding about their feelings and behaviours as their weight approaches or is within the normal weight range. In these sessions the aim is to help the woman continue to escape from the preoccupation with weight gain and food that she had when she was ill, and help her cope with life stress and other problems which may arise, without resorting to her previous disordered eating behaviour.

Continuing therapy may have to be available for many years. This means that the woman may need to know that she can contact her therapist and make an appointment or a series of appointments even if she has not had treatment for months or years.

Death due to anorexia nervosa gets newspaper headlines, particularly if a celebrity such as Karen Carpenter is the victim. However, fewer than 3 per cent of patients die from the effects of the eating disorder (half of whom die following a drug overdose). In short-term studies, predominantly of adolescent women, the death rate is 0–2 per cent. Long-term studies, which include the 20 per cent of chronic anorexia nervosa sufferers, suggest that up to 6 per cent of these patients will die over a period of years. However, with a greater community awareness about anorexia nervosa so that victims seek help earlier in the illness, and more physicians trained to manage the illness, the death rate is decreasing and is likely to be lower in the next decade.

Summary of treatment of anorexia nervosa

* Clinically not seriously ill
* Previous hospital treatment

* Severely ill on clinical examination
* Failure of outpatient or day-patient treatment
* The woman expresses a preference

↓   ↓

————Evaluate biochemical status————

↓   ↓

Usually treat as an outpatient
or as a day-patient
Other suggestions and support to
help patient:

Usually admit to
hospital
Provide programme to help patient:

* increase weight slowly by 0.3–0.5 kg (0.5–1lb) a week
* stop using weight-losing behaviour
* learn sensible eating patterns

* increase weight by 1–1.5 kg (2–3lbs) a week
* cease weight-losing behaviour
* learn sensible eating patterns
* exercise appropriately for body weight

↓

If the above goals are not achieved,
usually admit to hospital

Throughout programme provide:
* supportive psychotherapy
* cognitive and behaviour therapy
* help for other perceived problems (marital, family, medical)
* help in learning sensible eating patterns appropriate to lifestyle and age
* help in developing sensible exercise patterns
* confidence in ability to eat sensibly

↓

Later provide help for patient:
* to stabilise weight in desirable range
* to continue to avoid dangerous weight-losing methods
* to decrease preoccupation with weight and food
* to improve her self-esteem and self-concept so that it no longer depends on her body weight and shape

↓

Overall aim is to help:
* to live a normal life
* to be able to cope with life

10
Bulimia nervosa

I think that I look forward to a binge-eating session. Exactly what I am thinking is vague, but on reflection it is: 'Oh good, I won't have to think about dieting any more—what a relief.' If anything happens which delays the start of the binge I become quite angry and rather rude to the person who caused the delay. This anger is not warranted and is totally inappropriate—it could be likened to a temper tantrum.

Originally considered an 'ominous variant' of anorexia nervosa, bulimia nervosa is now accepted as being a separate eating disorder, although the two disorders have some features in common, particularly if the patient has the binge-eating and purging type of anorexia nervosa. Table 7, on p. 33, shows the accepted diagnostic criteria for bulimia nervosa.

Before the onset of bulimia nervosa, nearly all sufferers, when they were between the ages of 15 and 24, have had periods when they severely restricted their food (severe dieting), fasted, or resorted to 'fad' or 'crazy' diets. This in turn led to episodes of binge-eating when the woman's control over her food intake weakened. Over time the frequency and severity of the binge-eating increased and bulimia nervosa developed.

The prevalence of bulimia nervosa in the community amongst adolescent and young adult women, based on the strict criteria proposed by the American Psychiatric Association, indicate that the prevalence is 1 to 3 per cent. The true prevalence may be higher as only those women who seek medical help are identifiable. Even these women may not be diagnosed as bulimic. Most do not tell their doctor about their eating habit and, as a result, are investigated for gastro-intestinal problems, such as the irritable bowel syndrome (spastic colon), or gynaecological problems, such as infertility and menstrual disturbances, or are thought to be depressed and are given antidepressants. In the past the majority of binge-eaters only received help because of an excessive weight gain (or a weight loss) or because of an attempt at suicide, but now, because of articles in women's magazines, many women who have bulimia nervosa seek help earlier.

Case history: Jill

When I was 15, I looked at myself and thought: 'I'm too fat, and hate the size of my thighs and bottom'. My weight was then 63 kg (139 lbs, 9 st 13 lbs; BMI 23). So I started to diet taking in only 5040 kJ (1200 kcals), and got my father to buy an exercise bike which I rode for an hour each day. I lost 5 kg (11 lbs) of weight. In the next year I exercised a lot but ate normal meals and didn't gain weight. Then I got hepatitis and was in hospital for six weeks when my weight dropped to 54 kg (119 lbs, 8 st 7 lbs; BMI 20), but it built up to 57 kg (126 lbs, 9 st; BMI 21) in a few months—and that's the weight I think I look best at. So I was happy.

I went to 'Tech' when I was 18 and had a permanent boyfriend. We got on well but I started eating more and exercising less and my weight went up to 60 kg (132 lbs, 9 st 6 lbs). He said I was getting fat and so did May, a girl in the class who was really fat. I don't know if it was what they said, but about then I began to be very aware of women's bodies, and how much they varied in shape. I began to be quite obsessed with body shape and how it was often out of proportion and ugly and I began to diet to get my body into a better shape. It didn't do much good because my body remained the same shape and I didn't lose any weight although I tried for a year. I think I became convinced that I couldn't eat as much as other people because if I did I would get really fat like May.

Then my boyfriend and I split up and I was sure it was because I was fat. I started taking slimming pills—I suppose I took more than 20 of them some days. They didn't work either, so I tried I don't remember how many diets. I tried staying awake all night because I'd read that mental activity helped lose weight. I went to a doctor who gave injections to dissolve fat, but that didn't work either. I tried wearing plastic to lose weight. I tried hypnotherapy. And once, when I had 'flu I stood under a cold shower and then went outside in winter for two hours to try and catch pneumonia. I even stopped taking vitamin tablets because I thought that there might be calories in the capsules. Nothing worked for me, and my weight stayed between 63 and 66 kg (139–145 lbs, 9 st 13 lbs–10 st 5 lbs; BMI 23–5). It was very discouraging.

I felt the only way that I could really lose weight would be to starve. And I did, but I got so hungry that when I had fasted for two or three

Case history: Jill (continued)

weeks, only drinking fluids, I would binge-out. I used to go out late at night and buy food or if I could, steal it. I tried to induce vomiting after the binge by sticking my fingers down my throat but I couldn't manage it so I started taking quantities of laxatives, and when, after a binge, my ankles were swollen, I would get diuretic tablets from the doctor. My eating was really out of my control.

In fact I saw several doctors but none of them seemed to think there was anything wrong with me. So one day I took a large quantity of aspirin—I can't remember how many—to try to draw attention that I needed help—I really did need help!

Three years later she wrote to the clinic:

Looking back I think that the reason I started binge-eating was because of my obsession with dieting which stemmed from the fact I didn't realize in the first place that I wasn't overweight but that I had inherited fatter legs and thighs than the average person.

Stressful life events

The onset of bulimia nervosa may also be associated with stressful life events, which are not related to the woman's concern about body image or weight. A domestic argument, illness or death in the immediate family, the stress of examinations, a change in job, breakdown of a relationship, divorce, or pregnancy may precipitate the first eating-binge. The age of the woman has a bearing on which of the life events will precipitate binge-eating. Family problems or failure to achieve independence from parents are more common precipitants if the woman is teenaged, while, above the age of 20, marital and relationship difficulties are more common. Many women who have bulimia nervosa have a normal personality and no detectable psychopathology but some patients have a personality disorder which results in the woman having difficulties in everyday living. It is unclear whether the personality characteristics of binge-eaters have any relevance to the development of the illness, as they occur among women who do not binge-eat. Personality factors may play an important part in the woman's ability to recover and remain free from her illness.

It is important to be aware that the life events or problems in day-to-day living, which were associated with the onset of binge-eating, may be different from those which occur during the continuation of the disorder. These facts may have a bearing on the treatment adopted.

Bulimia nervosa and depression

Women who have bulimia nervosa have a low self-esteem, a low opinion of themselves, so that they may have depressive symptoms. These findings have led to much controversy among physicians who treat bulimic patients as to whether bulimia nervosa is caused by depression or whether the fear of weight gain, the physical effects of binge-eating, and the use of dangerous methods of weight control, increase the anxiety and guilt of binge-eating and cause depressive symptoms.

A recent study supports the view that the person's distorted attitudes to eating and to body image lead to depression rather than that depression leads to bulimia nervosa. This concept receives further support from a study of teenage women in the USA in 1990 in which it was found that twice as many women were depressed compared with men of the same age. The authors reported that the adolescent girls' preoccupation with their body shape and weight accounted for the difference.

As we discussed on page 54, low levels of serotonin in the brain seem to increase the amount of food a person wants to eat. It is thought that the low level resets upwards the 'appetite' or satiety centres in the brain. The antidepressant drugs (such as fluoxetine and paroxetine) which selectively inhibit serotonin re-uptake by the tissues, and thus increase the level of serotonin in the brain, should decrease the urge to eat and particularly to binge. These drugs do reduce the frequency of eating binges, at least in the short term. They are effective both in women who are depressed and bulimic women who are not depressed. Bulimia nervosa patients are however no more likely to have a depressive illness than other women in the community.

Binge-eating and panic attacks

Panic attacks are identified by a feeling of agitation and panic that seems to occur for no reason. Some women who suffer from panic attacks and also have bulimia nervosa may use food to cope with the feeling of panic. These women have described to us that they begin stuffing food into their mouths as soon as the panic attack starts and then vomit quickly. They say that in this way they are able to get over the attack in two or three minutes.

The eating-binge

It is easy to convince yourself on the day after each binge that that was the last one, and as of today you are never going to binge again. Unfortunately the nausea and feeling of self-revulsion disappears after a few days, and before you know it, the idea of escape into a session of eating unlimited amounts of anything that takes your fancy gets hold of you again. This can be caused by boredom, anxiety, or just a desire to relax or escape for a while.

Most binge-eaters are secretive about their behaviour. Many prepare secretively for the binge or plan for it by hoarding food beforehand. During the binge, as well as 'raiding the fridge', the woman usually prepares simple meals for herself, but some women prepare and cook elaborate dishes such as biscuits, cakes, and casseroles. Some women buy food especially to eat during episodes of binge-eating. About half eat most of their food during a binge in cafés or milk-bars, or go from shop to shop and to fast-food outlets buying food and eating it immediately.

Most bulimia nervosa patients gulp their food quickly during an eating-binge, some stuffing food frantically into their mouth, often making a considerable mess, leaving empty, open cans around. Other women are careful to make no mess so that they may avoid being found out. The rate of eating during an eating-binge varies between individuals and between binges. If the woman knows that she will not be disturbed, she will eat more slowly, particularly if she knows she can induce vomiting without being discovered. In general the rate at which she eats becomes slower as the binge-eating episode proceeds.

The binge may start at any time of the day and end as suddenly, but about one-third of binge-eaters have specific times, such as weekends, when they begin to binge-eat.

Food eaten during an eating-binge

The amount of food eaten during an eating-binge varies considerably, and ranges from 3 to 30 times the amount of food usually eaten in one day. The 'pickers' eat less than the 'stuffers', many stuffers eating over ten times the amount of food that they would eat each day when not bingeing. This can provide a large amount of energy, exceeding more than 83 700 kJ (20 000 kcal) during days of 'bad binge-eating'. Those who eat large quantities of food are more likely to reach higher body weights, to use slimming tablets and diuretics, to prepare food for a binge, to eat all the food that is available, to eat inappropriate foods, to have nocturnal binges, and to binge anywhere. The 'stuffers' are more likely to use and abuse alcohol or marijuana and may make an attempt at suicide following the episode of binge-eating.

Many binge-eaters claim they go on eating until they have eaten all the food available. But when this claim is analysed it is found that they are usually referring only to what they describe as 'binge' or 'bad' foods. They define these as foods they do not allow themselves to eat at other times, for example, cakes and ice-cream, peanuts, or biscuits. Only a few actually eat everything in the cupboards and fridge. By the time that most bulimia patients seek treatment, they either induce vomiting, or take purgatives, or both. This behaviour may take place during the binge or immediately the binge ends.

Why a binge-eating episode ends

The binge-eating episode ends for a variety of reasons. Some binge-eaters say simply that they 'ran out of steam'. Others stop because they feel discomfort being nauseated or full. Others because they can no longer continue to binge secretively.

After the binge, most binge-eaters promise themselves that they will keep to their strict diet or will fast and will not repeat the binge. A few fall asleep, but most take up their usual activities as if the binge had never happened.

Once binge-eating has been recognized by other people, most binge-eaters admit to it and some of them occasionally indulge in binge-eating in front of family members or close friends. A few binge-eaters use this in a manipulative way against parents or husband, implying: 'look what you have made me do'. Others go to great lengths to disguise their behaviour for long periods and are successful for many years. When discovered, most patients will admit to binge-eating and nowadays will usually admit to self-induced vomiting, if they use this method to control their weight. This is a recent change, probably resulting from the availability of information in non-medical publications about bulimia nervosa.

The duration and frequency of an eating-binge

It is difficult to be certain what bulimia nervosa sufferers mean by the length of a binge-eating episode, but it usually lasts for less than two hours. Women, especially those who have only recently developed abnormal eating behaviour, perceive their binge-eating as occurring in separate episodes, the number of binges on any one day of binge-eating ranging from one to six. Some women continue to binge-eat at this frequency. Other women, who frequently have a long history of binge-eating, may perceive their bingeing as occurring in discrete episodes, but having 10 to 20 episodes, a day, each being terminated by self-induced vomiting. Other women, again usually those with a long history of binge-eating, describe episodes lasting for days or weeks. By this they mean that the urge to binge-eat is continuous and is present even when they go to sleep and on waking, although it is obvious that they do not binge-eat continuously.

These descriptions of binge-eating given by women who have bulimia nervosa appear to differ from the criteria for bulimia nervosa of the American Psychiatric Association, but discussion with the woman will clarify the nature of her disorder.

Some women who are thought to have bulimia nervosa say that they only binge twice a month. These women do not have bulimia nervosa, as a diagnosis of bulimia nervosa can only be made if the woman binge-eats more than twice a week and has done this for at least three months. However they may have the binge-eating disorder or what the American Psychiatric Association has called an 'eating disorder—not otherwise specified (EDNOS)' and the World Health Organization an 'atypical eating disorder' (see Table, p. 39).

A physiological reason for binge-eating has been suggested. Normally when a person has eaten a normal amount of food, messages from her brain 'turn off' her desire to eat more. As most bulimia patients starve or diet strictly between eating-binges, they are in a 'food-deprived state' and changes in brain chemistry occur. One possible mechanism is discussed on page 50. When a person in a food-deprived state starts eating, the brain messages which normally 'turn off' appetite fail to work so that the person continues eating and overeats, commencing an eating-binge.

Food preference in bulimia nervosa

Each of the binge-eaters we have heard about or have studied include food in their binges which they do not allow themselves to eat at other times, calling them 'junk food', 'fat food', 'fattening food', or 'bad food'. Food eaten during a binge is sometimes selected because it is easy to 'stuff down' at the beginning of a binge, and easy to vomit up. Some of our binge-eaters said that their binges consisted mainly of soft, milky, or fluid foods, whereas others said they used such foods merely as a means to assist vomiting, and ate them towards the end of the binge.

The amount, type, and nutritional content of food eaten during a binge varies widely both within and between individuals. Contrary to most binge-eaters' impressions that the food eaten during binges is exceptionally high in fat, analysis of records of food actually consumed in a binge revealed that they were just as likely to contain excessive amounts of carbohydrate or protein. A few patients become vegetarian in order to control their weight and change from binges of food which are high in fat content to binges of fresh vegetables, on occasions, for example, eating 2–3 kg (4$^{1}/_{2}$–7 lbs) of raw carrots in a day. The amount, type, and nutritional content of food eaten during a binge may be entirely dependent on what is available in the home (Table 27). Some women will eat anything that is available, including tinned food, baby food, frozen food, and scraps from rubbish bins.

Precipitants of an eating-binge

There seem to be a number of factors which may precipitate an eating binge in a susceptible person. Most women say that before starting a binge they are unduly tense. Three-quarters say that loneliness or boredom precipitated a binge or that constant thoughts of food and a craving to eat, which they were eventually unable to control, were factors. Although many women diet rigidly between binges, only one-third say that hunger precipitates the binge.

A scenario might be that as the women are constantly concerned about their body image and keep to a diet to reduce their perceived ugly shape, an episode of loneliness, unhappiness, or boredom triggers thoughts of the pleasure of the taste of food, and this leads to an eating binge. Another possibility is that the woman finds that when she feels anxious or tense, the tension is relieved by binge-eating. This may occur because she inaccurately interprets her feeling of anxiety or tension as hunger.

Strategies used by bulimia nervosa sufferers to control weight

Women who have bulimia nervosa are aware that obesity is inevitable if they continue to binge-eat and do not take measures to control their weight. Their fear of fatness is as great as their love of food. Faced with this dilemma, two strategies are available to them. The first is to reduce the amount of energy absorbed from the food they eat by inducing vomiting during and after binge-eating and between binges. The second method is to diet strictly between binges. Some women choose to vomit as a strategy, others choose to diet. In addition to these primary measures, many binge-eaters in both groups use other methods of weight control, most of which are potentially dangerous. Between 75 and 90 per cent of binge-eaters abuse laxatives during a binge, at the end of a binge, or between binges. The reasons are twofold. First, purgation clears out the mass of 'bad' binge-food and the patient believes that it will prevent the energy being absorbed and converted into fat. Second, the use of purgatives relieves the fullness of abdominal discomfort and bloating which occurs after binge-eating. The quantities of purgatives taken varies from double the recommended dose, taken immediately after an eating binge, to 30 tablets, or 'handfuls' of laxative tablets every day. The prolonged

Table 27. Food eaten during a 'bad day' of binge-eating over a period of eight hours

3 loaves, 5 lb potatoes (chips), 1 jar honey, 1 jar anchovies (on bread),
1 lb rolled oats, 2 lb flour (as pancakes), 1 lb macaroni, 2 instant puddings,
4 oz nuts, 2 lb sugar, 1 large pkt Rice Bubbles, $1^{1}/_{2}$ lb margarine, 1 pint oil (for cooking), 4 pints milk powder, 1 tin condensed milk (in porridge, on bread or in drink), 4 lb ice-cream, 1 lb sausages (or meat rissoles), 1 $1^{1}/_{2}$ lb onions,
12 eggs (in milk-shake, scrambled eggs), 1 lb liquorice (liquorice allsorts),
2 family-size blocks chocolate, 1 lb dried figs, 2 pkts sweets, 6 'health bars',
assorted cream cakes (up to 12) eaten while shopping, 1 lb sultanas
(on bread or in porridge), left-overs found in fridge, 1 bottle orange cordial

This amount of food gives a total of:	
Energy	226 070 kJ (54 000 kcals)
Protein	1071 g
Fat	1964 g
Carbohydrate	14 834 g

regular use of laxatives to control weight gain amongst bulimia nervosa patients is declining in popularity as women are learning how ineffective they are in controlling body weight.

About 60 per cent of binge-eaters take commercial slimming 'pills', which contain some form of laxative, and a number take appetite-suppressing medications which may have an addictive property.

About 40 per cent of binge-eaters take large quantities of diuretic tablets, as they believe that the tablets will enable them to lose weight. Some women are aware that only fluid is lost, others believe that diuretics in some way 'dissolve' fat. And 10 per cent of binge-eaters abuse alcohol or drugs.

Case history: Karen

I find it easy to pinpoint the beginning of my illness. It began with an experience concerning one of my fifteenth birthday presents: a box of chocolates. I was at an age where pressures for social acceptance were, to me, immense, and pencil thinness, to me, was a prerequisite for social acceptance and self-confidence. I ate some of my birthday chocolates and was offered a suggestion by my mother; 'If you don't want to get fat, stick your fingers down your throat'.

Maybe this statement has more relevance than I'd previously thought. Mum's simple statement triggered off every emotional fear within me: 'I'll be fat—socially unacceptable—ugly—have no self-confidence—no self-esteem . . .' The fears were inexpressibly greater than I can even imagine now. My future, with those chocolates in me, appeared what can be plain and simply described as 'black'. My mother's suggestion seemed the only exit from the 'black future' I had prescribed for myself.

Naively I took this exit, which turned out not to be an exit at all but an entrance into hell. If only I'd known!

To induce vomiting was a revolting experience to me, but the fear of the 'black future' provided no alternative at all. Physical weakness and psychological euphoria followed my regurgitation. No matter how painful, or revolting, I'd found the key to freedom from that dreaded 'black future'.

I left school on my fifteenth birthday and found an increase in life's pressures. Coping became difficult, but I still possessed my 'key' to confidence and acceptance. I made a habit of vomiting after every evening meal and, as the months progressed, I gradually lost weight, believing that I was becoming more attractive all the while.

Case history: Karen (continued)

The fact that my food output by means of regurgitation was almost equal to my food intake allowed me to indulge for longer periods of time in my means of relief from life's pressures—eating—without gaining weight.

I became increasingly aware of my increasing ability to relieve life's pressure through the intake of food. Although the induction of vomiting continued to be traumatic, the relief beforehand, and the euphoria afterwards, were, to me, of no comparison to it. The vomiting became more frequent as the food intake rose and I accompanied my physically strenuous job with all the exercise I could muster. Some nights I could not sleep due to the immense guilt of either not having done enough exercise or having allowed too much food to digest.

By the age of 16 I found myself unable to cope not only with problems, but with spare time. Anxiety seemed to rule my existence and I could not relax without food. If, even then, I was relaxing, I'm unsure.

I felt revoltingly fat and ugly when I could not see all of my ribs when I looked in the mirror. I took a large daily dose of Epsom salts, along with what progressed to 13 laxative tablets daily.

Fortunately, my weight only regressed to just below 51 kg (112 lbs, 8 st; BMI 18) at its lowest. But it took its toll on my life. For breakfast I would eat 8–10 slices of toast plus cereal. Then I would do the dishes, eating everyone's scraps in an anxious, embarrassed, hidden hurry. I would then disappear inconspicuously to the toilet, and bring up my breakfast. My nose often bled, as did my stomach, and ten minutes later (to the dot) I would become very weak, dizzy, and pale.

I suffered malnutrition to the extent that my menstrual periods ceased for six or seven months. My god, I accepted such as being normal!!

During the following year, I began to realize that I was too thin so I fought my conscience and established my weight at about 57 kg (126 lbs, 9 st; BMI 20).

My eating, cunning and impatient as it was, had increased during this time, and I was spending about $A10 [£5] per day on food outside the house. This was quite substantial to me, for I was earning only $A120 [£60] per week. Fortunately I didn't have to pay board.

It was about this time that my boyfriend became too heavy to pursue his career as a jockey. I worried about his future, I worried about myself, I worried about everything and my only relief was food.

Case history: Karen (continued)

Being immature and mixed up, I acted strangely and desperately. My boyfriend had become part of a new group of friends who were heavily involved with drugs of every description—from heroin, to magic mushrooms, to petrol, and glue sniffing. This was beyond my capacity to cope. My 'other half' was dying and I was dying with him.

I knew subconsciously that I couldn't go on with him, nor could I go on without him. Without directly breaking up our relationship I acted in a manner which drove him and me 'up the wall'. I was subconsciously hoping that he'd break off our relationship and therefore I'd have it easier. It didn't work that day. He clung on, as I did. My eating worsened, my mind and soul weakened. He got deeper into the drug scene, and I began to follow, but, thank god, he loved me enough to keep me out of that 'black hole'. I suppose I'd have gotten in elsewhere if I'd really wanted to, but although I got drunk a couple of times and tried a few drugs, they did nothing for me. Food was my relief—my drug!

I isolated myself with food as often as possible. My crazy desperate behaviour dared, and received, the punishment it deserved. And one desperate day when I'd driven my boyfriend so hard he hit me and threw me down in the middle of the road (I was trying to stop him going to the pub), I returned to his house, alone and desperate. There was no food in the house, I had no money, and I felt that I could take no more of the torture I felt the world was inflicting upon me. I took a loaded shot-gun from the wall, and placed the end of the barrel in my mouth. I mustn't have wanted to die, because I received a sensation of strength which took away my need to pull the trigger. Although I didn't want to die, the desperation remained. I screamed and bashed the wall and cried for what must have been about an hour. After this I felt terribly weak. I returned to work but wouldn't speak to my boss, nor later to my family. They had no idea—nor did I want them to. I'd constructed an impermeable barrier around myself. I couldn't cope outside of it.

The next day I penetrated my barrier and began to feel my way into the world again, like a child's first adventure into a garden. I felt I had a new lease of life, when crash, down fell my depression and desperation, taking on a new tighter grip of me. I desperately ate my way through the day, resenting everyone and everything, playing sad music and feeling sorry for myself (although I didn't recognise self-pity then), and topping off the mountain of hate I had constructed against the world; or was it myself? I rather believe the latter.

I tried to escape. I went to Scotland and ate my way through my short stay there. I returned home and couldn't cope with a single day.

Case history: Karen (continued)

To my parents' horror and disappointment, I quickly packed and moved. The torture followed me, pouncing on me which ever way I turned. I spent my time obliviously eating my way through each day. Trying to live, but to no avail. At weekends I'd try to get home simply for the sake of the available food. I'd eat Mum out of house and home and the self-hate and guilt built up more and more due to my reasons for going home. It hurt me terribly when my mother confronted me with the fact that she was aware of my attraction to home. I loved my family dearly, but I then felt like a leech, so I went home as little as possible.

I spent my evenings at the local shops, with immense fear of being caught there, and with the guilt and anxiety continually mounting. To be so totally out of control in sobriety seemed so terribly degrading.

I couldn't cope with this life, so after five-and-a-half years of bingeing and vomiting I told my sister what I was doing. She arranged for me to see a doctor, who laughed at me and said 'What do you want me too do about it? Sew your mouth up?' I was temporarily numbed by this experience. The guilt and embarrassment then came on hot and strong, and I broke down crying in front of him. He then decided that I was crazy so he referred me to a psychiatrist.

She made me feel more acceptable to myself. Nevertheless, my obsession with food continued to increase. I couldn't bear to live with myself, so my psychiatrist arranged for me to be admitted to hospital as I wasn't improving.

If ever I've believed in my own 'God', it's now, for by what to me is a miracle, I've been identified as an addict, and have progressed to 12 days in a row without over-eating or vomiting. I hadn't succeeded through one single day in over a year before this, and how I'd tried!!

With the aid of the addiction program, and Alcoholics Anonymous philosophies, I've learnt more about myself and how to cope with life in the past 12 days than I have in the 20 years preceding. I'm gaining confidence, hope and see life as I've only dreamed of seeing it. I have a long way to go to recovery and I accept this. I've told the truth to my family and close friends, who have accepted it well. I'm truly getting there, and I won't give in for I've too much to lose. I've now had a taste of how enjoyable and exciting life can be; so hopefully I will be able to stay in the life I love so much, and hopefully maintain self-control for the rest of my life over my eating and vomiting.

How do binge-eaters try to resist binge-eating?

Nearly every binge-eater has attempted, at times, to resist the urge to binge. The methods chosen to resist the urge to binge-eat vary considerably. Some women feel a reduced urge if they keep no food in the house, buying only what is needed each day; others avoid cooking or going into the kitchen. Still others spend a long time chewing a mouthful of food to prevent themselves stuffing more and more food into their mouths. Other women avoid eating with the family or going out to social gatherings where food is served. A few women take more positive action by locking themselves in the bathroom, driving into the country where no food is available, or keeping no money in their purse. Still others try to divert their thoughts from food, planning to be completely occupied at all times, by knitting obsessionally, telephoning friends, or going out to meet people. Another method used by some women is to start doing jigsaw puzzles. After a few days of not binge-eating, the woman may feel very agitated. These feelings usually lead to her going to the kitchen and starting an eating binge. If a large jigsaw puzzle is on a table she may choose to go to the table and put in a few more pieces, rather than going to the kitchen and binge-eating. It appears that although she is unable to concentrate on reading or watching television, she may become absorbed by doing the jigsaw puzzle until the agitation passes. Some women undertake work with long periods of overtime, in jobs where no food is available; others try to keep to strict diets, or eat only minute quantities of food at a time and avoid food shops. Other women use exercise as a way of avoiding binge-eating. They spend long hours at the gym, play squash, or tennis, or run many miles every day. Ellen was one of these women who exercised to avoid binge-eating. She wrote:

The running was a great help to me in overcoming my eating problems and increasing self-esteem. I reached the point where going fast was more important than looking good, and of course an athlete has to eat well to race well. There is an overemphasis (I think) on skinfold measurements in endurance sports, however mine were always acceptable if not outstanding, without dieting.

Also, I think the ability to be aggressive in training and racing, and to push my body to its limits provided an outlet for the tension and anxiety that I used to release as bulimia.

I must admit to the occasional bulimic episode, perhaps once or twice a year. There are other times when I feel like it, but don't have the time or opportunity. These times are usually when I am angry but unable to express it; or feel out of control of my life or my time; or feel anxious or depressed. I think anger usually has something to do with it—again, I guess running was a good outlet for aggression, since when I was racing regularly the thought never entered my mind.

I still do not cope very well with putting on weight. I gained about 3 kgs during the first year (due to relative inactivity), but lost it quickly after the exams (lots of sport). I felt quite uncomfortable, physically and psychologically, at that weight. I wish it didn't matter to me, but it still does. However, I don't feel out of control, because I know that I can lose it easily.

Some women may try to avoid eating binges by abusing alcohol or other drugs. Other women abuse alcohol or drugs and continue binge-eating and vomiting. A few women who develop a drug or alcohol problem may recover from their eating disorder, but the drug or alcohol problem may persist for years and require treatment. One woman was so desperate she attempted to wire her jaws together by passing the wire through her gums after using a local anaesthetic ointment. Another cut the tips of her fingers so that they would be too sore to induce vomiting, hoping that this would stop her from starting on a binge.

Information about 'resistance behaviours' used by a binge-eater is often helpful in devising treatment.

The physical symptoms and signs associated with bulimia nervosa

Most compulsive eaters describe a number of physical symptoms associated with the binge. In addition, physical symptoms may follow induced vomiting or laxative abuse.

During an episode of binge-eating, most of the women feel 'bloated' or 'full' and some observe that their hands and feet swell. One-third are nauseated or complain of abdominal pain. By the end of the binge, over one-third complain of headache and half of the women complain of tiredness.

Self-induced vomiting

About six bulimia nervosa patients in every ten habitually induce vomiting. Initially vomiting is achieved by stuffing the fingers or a spoon into the throat, but later many women can induce vomiting by inducing a strong contraction of the diaphragm and abdominal muscles, to force the contents of the stomach into the oesophagus and then to vomit. In each episode of vomiting many women regurgitate one- to ten-times until they are certain all food has been brought up. Some women use 'markers', beginning a binge with food such as red apple skin, lettuce, or liquorice which they can recognize in the vomit. A number of patients also use 'wash-out techniques': they keep on drinking water and regurgitating until there is no residue of food in their stomach, a process which can last up to half an hour. In most cases the vomiting episodes last from 5 to 30 minutes, depending on ease of vomiting and quantity. In spit of these methods to insure vomiting is efficient, it does not prevent the absorption of foods, particularly the simple sugars that are absorbed quite quickly. To avoid detection they vomit into disposable containers or plastic bags. In one case the mother of the binge-eater habitually collected the vomited material and used it to fertilize the garden.

The physical effects of self-induced vomiting

Women who habitually induce vomiting may develop enlargement of their face and cheeks due to swelling of their salivary glands. Some

Table 28. The physical and psychological changes which may accompany bulimia nervosa

Fatigue
Lethargy
Mood disturbance
Anxiety symptoms
Abdominal discomfort
Constipation
Menstrual irregularity
Dry skin
Calluses on back of fingers (if a vomiter)
Dental enamel erosion leading to chipped, ragged, 'moth-eaten' teeth

women develop calluses on the back of their fingers as a result of inserting them frequently into their mouth to induce vomiting. Some women retain fluid after binge-eating large amounts of food and then inducing vomiting. This is especially disconcerting to a woman who is anxious about gaining weight. Most of the women who habitually induce vomiting have had extensive and expensive dental work to correct the damage to their teeth caused by acid vomit which etches away the tooth enamel. Over half of the women who induce vomiting often, report that sometimes the vomit contains blood.

Case history: Charlie
After a long illness Charlie recovered from anorexia nervosa. Her father wrote to thank us for the efforts we had made to help her recover. 'The cost of inpatient treatment was high', he wrote, 'but I do not begrudge that. What I do begrudge is the A$3000 that I had to pay to the dentist to repair the damage Charlie had done to her teeth. Before she became ill she had the most beautiful teeth. They will never be the same, even with the dental care they have received'.

Of greater danger to the women is that frequent self-induced vomiting over a period of time may result in dehydration and possible disturbances in the electrolytes in the blood, cardiac arrhythmias and changes in the electrocardiogram, renal problems, and occasionally death (see page 146).

When a woman stops vomiting she may suffer abdominal cramps, bloating, constipation or diarrhoea, and may feel exhausted or become very agitated. These 'withdrawal' symptoms cease after ten days. Three weeks later she is no longer agitated or fatigued and usually says that she feels better than she has done for years.

Laxative, slimming tablet, and diuretic abuse

Over 75 per cent of women have taken laxatives to purge themselves either during or immediately after the binge. In some cases the quantity of laxatives taken is considerable, ranging from twice the recommended dose to 'handfuls'. Many of the women are aware that the diarrhoea following excessive laxative intake may lead to electrolyte disturbances, particularly potassium deficiency, and avoid them by eating potassium-rich foods such as oranges or tomatoes. The use of laxatives is irrational as well as potentially dangerous. Laxatives act mainly on the large bowel inducing it to empty, but this occurs *after* the energy obtained from the food eaten has been absorbed in the small intestines. All that laxatives do is cause the body to lose fluid, not energy. This is followed by rebound water retention so that the person's body weight may be higher after taking laxatives than it was before.

Stopping laxative abuse is also followed by 'withdrawal' symptoms, which are similar to those which follow cessation of self-induced vomiting. These are constipation, abdominal cramps, abdominal bloating, agitation, and feeling 'awful'. A woman needs to be reassured that these symptoms, which usually occur, are normal, and will cease after ten days.

Half of patients who have bulimia nervosa have taken 'slimming tablets' or diuretics to lose weight, and these women may also abuse the diuretics with an inevitable electrolyte disturbance, particularly a potassium deficiency, unless they take measures to prevent this happening. As many of them are aware of the problems of potassium deficiency, they take potassium supplements or drink orange juice which is rich in potassium. In some cases severe potassium deficiency occurs which requires treatment in hospital.

Diuretics only rid the body of water and electrolytes: they do not have any effect on ridding the body of stored fat. Their regular use may lead to short-term, or long-term, persistent fluid retention when they are discontinued.

Menstrual disturbances

Many binge-eaters develop menstrual irregularities, although, in contrast to women who have anorexia nervosa, their body weight is usually in the normal range for age and height or they are slightly overweight. About 40 per cent of women who have bulimia nervosa develop irregular menstruation and, in another 20 per cent, menstruation ceases. Women who cease to menstruate may be found to have high levels of cholesterol in their blood, which may cause concern, but the levels tend to fall when menstruation returns. These women need reassurance that menstruation will become normal when their body weight stabilizes and when they have ceased to use dangerous methods of weight control, including intermittent starvation and excessive exercise.

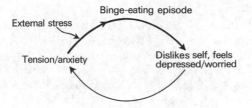

Fig. 15. The psychological circle of binge-eating.

The psychological effects of binge-eating

Before starting to binge-eat, most women feel tense and anxious, have palpitations, or begin sweating. During the binge, most binge-eaters feel a sense of freedom; the anxiety or worry they had been experiencing lifts and they no longer have anxious or negative thoughts. If the woman chooses to induce vomiting, she may also reduce tension with the act of vomiting. At the end of the binge, most binge-eaters feel less tense and anxious, but may not like themselves because of what they have done to their bodies. They may feel guilty about inducing vomiting and panic that the binge may induce a weight gain. This in turn may lead to further anxiety and tension, with the result that they may start binge-eating once again. A vicious circle is established (Fig. 15). The physical and psychological changes which may accompany bulimia nervosa are shown in Table 28.

If a binge-eater is unable to relieve her anxiety and tension, for example, if the person is interrupted or discovered when binge-eating, her behaviour may change to agitation, anger, or aggression.

It is also apparent that if a woman with bulimia nervosa does not recognize the tension and anxiety or has no other ways of coping with them, she easily enters the vicious circle and becomes a frequent binge-eater. As will be seen, a major objective of treatment is to break this vicious circle of eating behaviour.

Case history: Penny
I really started binge-eating when I was about 12. Before that I had bought lots of sweets, candies, and lollies, because Mum gave me a lot of pocket money—but all kids do that. Then, when I was about 12, I started dieting and began binge-eating. I remember that I used to eat

Case history: Penny

my pack lunch on the way to school and then scrounge food from the other kids. By the time I was 14, I was a real binge-eater. After a binge I would vomit and after a time I could vomit without putting my fingers down my throat. I still can, but I don't do it. What with study and fixing up bingeing, I didn't have time for friends. But it didn't seem to matter, I just had to binge-eat and I did, and then I vomited so that I wouldn't put on weight.

That went on until I was 20. I had this job—it was so boring and I hated it. One day after an eating-binge, I was so agitated I drank half a bottle of sherry. It worked wonders. It steadied my nerves and I felt better. I started thinking that if I had a drink I wouldn't need to binge-eat. I bought a bottle of whisky and kept it in my wardrobe. When thoughts of food and putting on weight became overwhelming I'd drink some alcohol and they would be less insistent. That's how I stopped bingeing. I went on vomiting—it's easy to do when you know how and my weight dropped from 67 kg (148 lbs, 10 st 8 lbs; BMI 26) to 46 kg (101 lbs, 7 st 3 lbs; BMI 18). When I was drinking I was much more relaxed and began to go out with friends.

About this time I realized I was wasting my life so I left the dull job and stopped drinking, except on social occasions when I would drink until I was drunk, or eat all the food I could. I guess the occasions gave me permission to indulge my needs. I started a secretarial course, which was hard work, and one day I began binge-eating again. It was just after my 21st birthday when I had got drunk and had horrified my parents. Soon I was binge-eating three or more times a week. I started vomiting again and took large doses of laxatives. Because I was scared that I would put on weight even after what I was doing, I began to jog and was soon running 6 miles (10 km) a day. It seemed to help. When I was jogging I stopped thinking about food and my weight, which stayed at 54 kg (119 lbs, 8st 7 lbs; BMI 21). Because of the vomiting my teeth were going bad, but I couldn't stop vomiting after an eating-binge; it made me feel relaxed. And if I was having problems, or was worried, I'd drop into the pub and have a few quick whiskys. Mind you, I was worried that I might be an alcoholic.

The next year I met Wayne and we married. It was great at first but I still needed to binge, and I did, often every day, and I kept a bottle or two of whisky hidden at home, just in case I needed a drink. When Wayne found out he was furious and I felt it was time I saw a doctor.

The Clinic records show that over the next three years, when Penny was attending regularly, she occasionally binge-ate and twice returned to her previous behaviour of binge-eating three or more times a week and using alcohol. Her weight is stable at around 55 kg (121 lbs, 8 st 9 lbs; BMI 21), and she leads an active social life. Her employer says she is excellent at her job.

The effect of bulimia nervosa on body weight

Before developing the eating disorder the body weight of most binge-eaters is within the normal range. About 20 per cent are overweight or obese, and a similar proportion are underweight, often being diagnosed as having anorexia nervosa. After starting the binge-eating, many of the women show frequent swings in body weight. These facts indicate that women of all weights may binge-eat. Binge-eating occurs among obese women, women of normal body weight, and some anorexia nervosa patients binge-eat.

Case history: Jane
Jane started dieting at the age of 16 to control her weight. At first she had a small steady loss in weight. At the age of 17 she began binge-eating and for the next six years she alternated between binge-eating and strict, almost starvation diets, with resulting large swings of weight, of up to 19 kg (42 lbs, 3 st). When her weight was below 55 kg (121 lbs, 8 st 9 lbs), her menstrual periods ceased, to return when her weight exceeded that weight. On two occasions of about two-weeks' duration her weight fell to a BMI of 15, placing her into the category of anorexia nervosa, as it is defined clinically.

Other binge-eaters control their weight fluctuations to within 3 kg (6½ lbs), by dieting and exercising excessively between binges, or by using vomiting and purging to try to prevent absorption of the food eaten during a binge. The belief held by many women who have bulimia nervosa that self-induced vomiting, immediately after eating, is a very efficient way of controlling weight gain as no food is absorbed, is erroneous. Some food must be absorbed, as women who binge-eat a large amount of food are usually overweight, whilst the weight of women whose binges are small is usually in the normal range.

The treatment of bulimia nervosa

The one major element required for recovery from bulimia is a desperate will to live normally. Normality is the heaven for which I strive. Perhaps I will have it some day. I certainly haven't given up. This however is not as simple as it sounds to a binge-eater. It should be so easy to forget about counting calories and just eat three normal meals every day, but somehow the reassurance of knowing that you didn't eat more than your allowed calories is necessary. Without this reassurance, confusion can result, bringing on a binge. Counting calories doesn't mean dieting or denying yourself fattening foods—it simply means controlling your overall food intake and allowing for these fattening extras in your diet. It can stop the guilt associated with eating high-calorie items, a guilt which may be the cause of a binge.

The wide variation in eating behaviours of binge-eaters, the changes which occur in an individual over a period of time, the symptoms associated with binge-eating, and the consequences which may arise indicate that treatment has to be individualized and should be aimed to help the particular individual correct her disordered eating behaviour.

Bulimia nervosa patients are frequently extremely demanding of time, and they may also be manipulative and not always truthful, as they are usually desperate for help and want the therapist to like them. Most do realize that their behaviour is abnormal so it is perhaps not surprising that they are not always truthful. However they have a number of assets which makes working with them rewarding for the therapist. Even though not always appropriate, the resources that they have developed, such as their behaviour to resist binge-eating and their desire to get better, mean that progress can be made once the therapist and the patient have formed a good, trusting relationship.

The aims of treatment

The aims of the treatment of bulimia nervosa are:

- to help the woman acquire new attitudes to food, eating, body shape, and weight;
- to help her reduce her preoccupation with food;
- to help her keep her weight in the normal range (BMI 19–24.9) or at an agreed weight above this range;
- to persuade her to eat a meal three times a day, with one or two snacks if she wishes;

- to help her avoid inappropriate methods for losing weight such as self-induced vomiting, laxative abuse, and compulsive exercise;
- to help her obtain insight into her mood changes and to learn to cope with these moods using ways other than binge-eating;
- to help her recognize what precipitates her binge-eating;
- to help her find ways to cope with her problems, other than resorting to binge-eating;
- to help her to improve her self-esteem.

The most successful treatment to date is cognitive-behavioural therapy. This involves a trusted therapist and a dietitian. Other health professionals, particularly skilled nurses, may be involved.

Cognitive-behavioural therapy CBT

Cognitive-behavioural therapy is described on page 116 (you might care to read that section before going on). Before starting on treatment the history of the eating disorder and the woman's physical condition is checked so that any specific needs can be addressed during cognitive-behavioural treatment. Some of these needs will be discussed later in this chapter. During the interview the therapist (or the dietitian) stresses the importance of keeping a mood diary and a food diary in the first weeks of treatment (see page 111). The therapist discusses the mood diary with the patient and helps her separate mood from food. In other words to help her discover that her moods and feelings are not dependent on whether she will eat, what she has eaten, whether she has dieted, or if she feels 'fat' and unattractive. The dietitian discusses the food diary with the woman and encourages her to stop weighing herself more than once weekly, counting kilojoules (calories), reading food labels cooking for others and reading recipes. Table 29 summarizes the details of the cognitive-behavioural treatment.

More recent studies of treatment suggest the time for formal cognitive-behavioural therapy can be reduced; six weeks for Stage I is equally beneficial and effective as longer times (Table 29). In practice Stage I and Stage II overlap. When a woman is completing her daily diaries and discussing these with her therapist, she gains insight into her behaviour and realises that some of her beliefs and fears are no longer valid. This allows her to change her behaviour.

Table 29. Cognitive-behavioural treatment—a summary

Preliminary
The therapist:
(1) takes a comprehensive history of the eating disorder, checks the patient's physical, reproductive (including menstrual), and psychological health, her family history, and explores her attitudes to her eating problem;
(2) establishes trust between the patient and herself, and introduces her to a dietitian.

Stage I—weeks 1–6 (meetings once or twice each week)
The therapist:
(1) persuades the patient to record in detail everything she eats, at what times she eats, and how much and what thoughts and feelings she has during eating. (The Food and Mood Diaries (Tables 17 and 18) may be chosen or one of the other records shown in the self-help manuals.) The recorded information is discussed at the weekly meetings;
(2) offers alternative behavioural choices to help the patient resist binge-eating
The therapist asks the patient to meet with the dietitian, who:
(1) persuades her to eat food at regular intervals and not to binge-eat;
(2) teaches her about food and eating behaviour.

Stage II—weeks 6–12
The therapist:
(1) helps the patient explore why she started binge-eating;
(2) helps her change her thoughts about problems with her eating behaviour, her shape, and her weight;
(3) helps her develop skills to deal with difficulties which trigger binges;
(4) discusses with the patient the role (if any) of family, partner, or social situations.
The dietitian:
(1) starts gradually introducing avoided or 'feared' (which the patient perceives as 'bad') foods into her diet;
(2) gradually eliminates all forms of strict dieting.

Stage III—weeks 12–24
At this stage most patients have not fully recovered. The therapist reassures the patient that progress will continue and reassures her that even when the programme finishes, help will be readily available if her symptoms return or worsen, or if she has any further problems.

With thanks to Christopher Fairburn for permission to paraphrase his summary of cognitive-behavioural therapy, which he has developed and tested since 1980.

Where should a patient with bulimia nervosa be treated?

When the diagnosis has been made and the patient's condition has been assessed, several approaches to treatment are available and should be discussed by the therapist and the patient.

The possibilities including the following.

- *Self-help using a self-help manual* (see Further reading). This approach may be chosen as an initial method by women who have concealed from their family that they have bulimia nervosa, and have chosen not to seek professional help. We believe, however, that an initial assessment by a trained therapist is a better choice.

- *Guided self-help.* The patient is first assessed by a health professional and then chooses to use a self-help manual. At intervals she returns to consult the health professional with whom she has established trust, so that she can discuss any problems which have arisen and can monitor progress.

- *Ambulant treatment.* This is usually provided by an eating disorders team. The team includes a psychiatrist or clinical psychologist and a dietitian. The woman's general practitioner may also become involved.

- *Day-patient attendance at a specialized Eating Disorder Unit.* The programme for day care is more extensive than that provided by ambulant care and may be the most appropriate choice for many women.

Some treatment centres conduct formal cognitive-behavioural therapy for groups of women with bulimia nervosa. A recent study suggests individual cognitive-behavioural therapy is slightly more effective. Taking an individual approach to therapy allows treatment to be planned to meet the needs of an individual woman, her stage of illness, her current beliefs and attitudes, her motivation to change, and the external difficulties or stressors that may be preventing her recovery. To make day programmes more effective a combination of group and individual therapy can be provided.

Interpersonal therapy IPT

The effectiveness of interpersonal therapy was found by accident. It was compared with cognitive-behavioural therapy in a very well conducted study of treatments conducted in Oxford in the United Kingdom. Interpersonal therapy in this study was designed to provide a treatment, instead of no treatment, and a treatment as different to CBT as possible. It was hoped that this would show the effectiveness of CBT in the treatment of bulimia nervosa. In this study inter-personal therapy consisted of the therapist and patient discussing and producing aims for therapy, for example, to improve self-esteem, but there was to be no discussion about matters relating to eating and body weight or shape. The therapist remained supportive, neutral, and non-directive throughout each session. In the first few months, not surprisingly, cognitive-behavioural therapy was significantly more effective than interpersonal therapy; the women's attitudes to weight and shape were more improved. After one and five years both were equally effective and significantly more effective than a third group who did not receive CBT or IPT. This suggests that the long-term outcome of therapy does not depend on therapy being aimed at eating and body image concerns.

Combined therapies

The ideal approach is to assess each woman individually and evaluate the possible usefulness of the various therapies for the woman; nutritional therapy, antidepressant medication (SSRI's), cognitive-behavioural therapy, interpersonal therapy, stress reduction, family or marital therapies. Any combination of these can be employed at the same time or at different stages of treatment. In clinical practice a combination of approaches is used, particularly if treatment is provided by a team of people trained in different disciplines. Studies of treatment involving a combination of therapies are showing promising results. The advantage is that if the programme is scheduled for weekends or for 2–3 days a week the woman can continue working part-time. There are problems, however. Some women use manipulative behaviour, such as threats of suicide, to gain admission to hospital when facing personal, work, or other challenges.

- *Hospital treatment.* Treatment in hospital has the advantage of enabling a lot to be accomplished in a short period of time. The woman has the opportunity to take part in small group therapy, learn social skills, assertiveness training, psychodrama, and anxiety management.

However, in most cases, hospital admission and in-patient treatment is undesirable in the first instance, unless the woman is in 'crisis' or has severe psychological, psychiatric, or medical problems such as depression, or is suicidal, or has a severe personality disorder (Table 30).

The reason is that some in-patients take on the role of a psychiatric patient (in many cases patients with an eating disorder are treated in a psychiatric unit). They avoid responsibility for changing their own behaviour, expecting the hospital staff to take on this responsibility.

For this reason women who are admitted to hospital tend to have severe symptoms, or have multiple psychological or physical problems. This may be the reason why hospital treatment seems to be no more successful than out-patient treatment in effecting a cure.

Other reasons for hospital admission include women whose out-patient treatment has not been successful over a six or twelve month period; women whose life is in crisis and may benefit from a short stay in hospital, so that her therapist can assess her medical and psychological problems and devise a treatment programme which is appropriate for the woman. Hospital admission may also be necessary for a woman who lives in a country area which prevents her from attending as an out-patient.

In the Eating Disorders Unit at which Suzanne Abraham is Co-Director, the in-patient treatment programme is intensive and involves the patient being in contact with a range of people from different health disciplines. Each patient has her own special nurse

Table 30. Possible reasons for admitting a patient with bulimia nervosa to hospital

If she is in poor physical health because she uses dangerous methods of weight control

If she has medical, psychological, or psychiatric problems which are best treated in hospital (for example, depression, drug addiction, severe biochemical disturbance, personality disorder)

If she is suicidal

If her home environment is preventing changes in her eating behaviour

If her personality is such that our-patient treatment is unlikely to be effective

If she lives in a remote area where out-patient treatment is not available

If no improvement has been obtained as an outpatient, particularly if several attempts have failed who co-ordinates the programme and acts as an advocate between the formal sessions with her psychiatrist or psychologist.

The problems experienced by some women who require admission to hospital are graphically illustrated by the following extracts from the diary of a 19-year-old patient, called Erin, who was both popular with her peers and outstanding in her studies before she acknowledged the need for treatment.

Erin's Diary, Week one

First, I must accept the fact that it is my problem and, even if it isn't all my fault, I am the one who has to do the work to cure it . . . and not play games . . .

I need to give some time to myself to think about my problem. I have to stop trying to keep busy to stop trying to take my mind off the problem and to stop the loneliness.

I'm thinking about packing up and leaving and sorting it out at home instead of here . . .

I want to know more about my problem:
— why has it happened?
— what happens to me?
— what I need to get better . . . ?

I wish there were some rules to follow to get better, it's so hard because it is not a physical problem: it's emotional and psychological . . .

The one cause or associated problem is my fear of being alone, which I find hard to understand and which is pretty paradoxical. I'm afraid of being left alone at home or out because I know that I'll lose control and binge-eat. On the other hand, when I'm feeling like binge-eating, I get irritated when somebody is with me because they are preventing me from starting the binge. That is the paradox I'm beginning to understand . . .

The anxieties that started me binge-eating have long since passed I think. Now the bingeing is habitual and creates anxieties instead of the anxieties creating the binge. The anxieties that are created by the loss of control, and the binge, and the low self-esteem that goes with it, cause the bingeing behaviour. I'm not sure how to correct this but think that it has some relevance—there's more to it as well I'm sure . . .

End of week one

God, where do I start? I'm really so confused . . . there's so much to grasp at once.

I'm constantly trying to please people and to do what I believe they expect of me and *I have stopped being myself* because of it. Always being ready to listen to and to help others. Always being *selfless* is partly a cause of this problem.

Week two

I've been very moody and restless since Wednesday. Woke up OK today but since breakfast I've been really angry. Stuffed myself with AllBran and feel revolting and fat. Just want to throw it up—now I know that anger leads to purging: anger, self disgust, revulsion and hatred . . .

End of week two

Still angry and frustrated and confused. All day I felt dreadful . . . felt fat and ugly and dreadfully alone and empty. I cried, being so angry and frustrated and not understanding what was going on. I was ultra-upset after my appointment with the dietitian. She made it clear to me just how I've been stuffing myself around by cutting back on my menu plan. Losing 750 g while cutting back—which is pretty easy to do in here because you don't build up much appetite—is stupid. To cut back while being in here is stupid because the minute I go out I'll cut back, deny myself things and then binge and vomit and be back to square one. It's just so futile! All I want to do is lose weight and get over this eating disorder. I have to *stop cutting back*, which means stop losing weight . . .

End of week three

I want to go home. But I know that's running away. But it won't really be running away. I'll be running away from *this environment to another environment, but the feelings* won't change. *I can run away as far as possible, but I can't run away from how I'm feeling.*

Oh, what a day! YUCK . . . YUCK . . . YUCK . . . ! [later] The *best thing* I did for myself tonight was to stop myself from bingeing and *I feel so good* about it.

On my way to bed I stuffed my pockets with about 15 biscuits, but after eating four (*I think I was so off the planet with mixed emotions I'm really unsure*) I came back to my room and my positive—very positive *new mind* defeated the bingeing.

I thought '*Be nice to yourself—do something good for yourself for a change*', and I picked up all the biscuits and took them and got rid of them. I felt so *powerful.* I jumped for joy and happiness about myself . . .

End of week four

Some nights when I have the urge to binge I don't go near the kitchen, I feel strong and those times are positive. But tonight's defeat of the

Bulimic Binge Devil was even stronger. Stronger because I'd taken the first step and there was *no chance* of being caught.

I'm so *pleased*, because that's the hardest thing I've done for a long time. And the best thing was that *I did it for myself. For nobody else but me and I did it for me*

because
I
deserve
to
beat
it.

Week five

Went home on Friday. Aaaaaaarghhhh! I'm going up and down like a yo-yo. It's unbelievable. I did vomit and then felt so *guilty*, mainly for Mum but also for myself.

End of week five

This morning I woke up with a new attitude. I realized last night that going home without taking responsibility just wasn't the answer. Responsibility for my own dilemma was the key to beating it. I made some decisions . . .

Spoke to my doctor which annoyed me because she emphasized the importance of getting on with it.

I can't FANTASIZE . . .
I must do it.

Continuing support and follow-up

The importance of continuing support from the therapist cannot be overemphasized, as relapses in the first two years of treatment may occur. If the woman has been treated in hospital and has been discharged, she may start binge-eating again within a few weeks or months. If she can readily contact her therapist or one of the skilled staff of the Eating Disorders Unit she can seek their help to avoid falling into this behaviour pattern.

If a day programme is available for one or two days a week, it may provide the support needed. A weekend programme can allow the woman to return to study or work immediately after leaving hospital. A woman will find the transition much easier if she has to make only one change in her routine between being an in-patient and her normal daily pattern of living. For this reason, going on holiday or any other intermediate step between being in hospital and out-patient follow-up treatment is not recommended.

She should also be able to obtain skilled help, if a stressful life event occurs, such as the challenge of an examination or a new job, or if an interpersonal relationship ends, so that she can be helped through the crisis without resorting to bulimic behaviours.

During the time that a woman is suffering from bulimia nervosa, she should not take a part-time job which is associated with food, such as waitressing, because preparing or serving food is likely to provoke an episode of bulimia and to retard or prevent recovery. Similarly, jobs associated with exercise and body shape, such as becoming an aerobics instructor, may prevent recovery.

Until the woman has recovered from bulimia nervosa for at least six months, she should avoid long holidays or trips overseas. In an unfamiliar environment, with the loss of routine, frequent new experiences, and different foods it is common for bulimia nervosa patients to feel that they have lost control of their body weight and to revert to a pattern of binge-eating, self-induced vomiting, and purgation. Because of the fear of returning to binge-eating and purging, some women recovering from bulimia nervosa respond by not eating and then become ill, with extreme weight loss, and need to return home quickly.

Changing attitudes to food, shape, and weight

In the back of my mind, I still feel that—should events one day go bad in my life—I could return to the bingeing as before. If there was too much pressure, worries, or if I couldn't cope with problems, food is the crutch to keep me going. It would have to be very bad, but I also think I would seek help from my counsellors to keep me from turning entirely to food. I'm not sure—it exists as a possibility. Certainly, if I was bored, unhappy with my lifestyle (for example, stuck in a little house with a baby and no friends or money to buy things) or doing things I did not really want to do—food or eating might become the only interesting facet of life (as they were once to me). But I hope not. And I think—I really think—I'll make it without food in the long run.

Women who have bulimia nervosa, like other people who have eating disorders, are preoccupied with food and the shape and weight of their bodies. They have to be encouraged to stop keeping food records, weighing themselves frequently, reading recipes, and cooking for others, as these behaviours prevent them recovering. On page 109 we mentioned the value of keeping mood and food diaries in the early weeks of treatment. The diaries can demonstrate to the woman that her episodes of binge-eating may have decreased, although she is not aware of this, or that while she is premenstrual and during early menstruation the eating binges may increase. This is a physiological response and does not mean that her progress is ceasing.

Bulimia nervosa sufferers should be encouraged to eat out socially and increase other social activities. Most of them have withdrawn from social occasions because of the presence of food or because of feelings of social unease, not related to food. They need help to find out what social eating is and to learn to incorporate it into their lifestyle. The fewer diet restrictions there are the easier this is. It also means giving up the distinction between 'good foods' and 'bad foods'.

'Good' and 'bad' foods

Bad foods are perceived by bulimia nervosa patients as foods which contain fat or are high in simple carbohydrates (sugars). In Table 31 we have listed foods our patients thought to be good or bad.

This table shows that many of the 'good' foods are those recommended by expert committees concerned about preventing heart disease, diabetes, and obesity. However, many eating disorder patients' ideas about foods are not accurate and the likelihood of a woman being able to resist eating all of the foods on the 'bad' list over a long period of time is very small. Learning to eat all foods in moderation at meal times or on social occasions, rather than only during binge-eating, is an important action for women who are recovering from bulimia nervosa to learn.

Normal and abnormal eating

The main treatment objectives are to help the bulimia nervosa sufferer change her thoughts about food, her body shape and weight, and to persuade her to eat normally. Many of these women have forgotten what normal eating is and need encouragement and help to change their thoughts about normal and abnormal eating. Tables 31, 32, and 33 may help them to achieve this objective.

Table 31. The perception of 'good' and 'bad' foods by women who have eating disorders

'Bad' foods	'Good' foods
Energy-dense foods	High fibre foods
Foods containing fat	Foods with no fat content
Take-away ('junk') foods, including	
hamburgers	Vegetables, but not potatoes
Snack foods	Fruit
Dairy products, including milk	
and cheese	Yoghurt (by some women)
Red meat	Chicken and fish
Bread and biscuits, cakes	Diet biscuits
Sweets, lollies, candies, chocolate,	Anything bought in a health
ice-cream	food shop, including honey

Case history: Maggie
The beauty of bulimia always seemed to be that I could eat as much as I wanted, because I knew I could get rid of it either through vomiting, exercise, laxatives, or starving. For the last six years, I have used food as my comfort whenever I felt angry, sad, anxious, bored, or felt any uneasy feeling. I knew food would make me feel better instantly. I would eat my favourite foods. I would buy them especially for a binge. Chocolates, Twisties, chips, cakes, lollies, pies, sausage rolls, cheese dips, and biscuits—all foods that I class in the 'bad food' category. I would eat until I felt better, but then I would start to feel bad again and my behaviours, like vomiting, would erase those bad feelings almost instantly.

I would say at the end of every binge: 'This is the last time I will ever do this', and I would go for days when I wouldn't eat anything. I would just drink water. Then I would eat things that I classed as 'good' foods—fruit, diet foods, vegetables, foods with the least amounts of calories and fat. Or maybe for a week I would just eat a chocolate bar every day.

But then I would build back up to a binge again. All the bad food would come back out again. Control was lost in every way. And I thought this was normal eating.

Table 32. Normal eating

Normal eating is:
- eating something at least three times a day, with snacks between as guided by one's appetite;

- eating a wide variety of foods as part of a balanced and flexible diet;

- eating more of the foods whose taste and texture you enjoy when you wish to;

- eating more than you feel the need to eat on some occasions (overeating);

- eating less than you need on some occasions (undereating);

- eating in a flexible way so that it does not interfere with your work, study, or social life, and vice versa;

- eating or not eating on occasions when you feel unhappy, 'bad', or tense;

- eating, when out socially, in a similar manner to the other people in the group;

- eating at fast food outlets occasionally when you wish to or are with your friends;

- being aware that eating is not the most important thing in life but that it is important for good health, physical and mental well-being;

- being able to prepare food for yourself and others without feeling anxious;

- knowing what portions of food and size of meals are appropriate in different circumstances.

Control of weight

As most bulimia nervosa patients have experienced large swings in body weight during the years of binge-eating, part of the treatment is to help the woman learn, often for the first time, how to stabilize her body weight and maintain it within the 'desirable' range. But first the woman and the therapist have to agree upon a sensible weight, which the patient will seek to maintain. This is because in some cases the woman may have to accept a weight which is higher or lower than the weight she desires to achieve. Evidence is becoming available which suggests that men and women who eat normally have an individual 'set point' for their body weight (and body fat). This set point, also called the adipostat or appetite/satiety centre is a network of neurones in the brain which serves to maintain a set amount of adipose body tissue for a particular body. If the person's weight is artificially low for her adipostat, her brain may respond in a way (for example, inducing hunger so that

Table 33. What normal eating is not

Normal eating is:
- *not* dieting;

- *not* counting calories (kilojoules), weighing food, or following a strict diet (unless medically indicated);

- *not* eating to lose weight, unless you are obese, but eating to remain in a stable weight-range appropriate for your body;

- *not* aiming to eat a diet containing no fat;

- *not* eating low energy substitute foods, e.g. diet biscuits rather than bread;

- *not* feeling when you eat a particular food you will be unable to stop until it is all eaten;

- *not* having to weigh yourself for reassurance;

- *not* avoiding eating because you do not know what the food contains;

- *not* playing games with yourself to prevent eating certain foods, e.g., saying to yourself 'dairy products make me feel nauseous';

- *not* being obsessed with food.

the person eats more) aimed at restoring her weight to the set point. Similarly if a woman has increased her body weight above her set point, the adipostat may be activated to reduce her hunger so that she eats less and loses some body weight. Women (and men) who have an eating disorder may 'inactivate' their adipostat in some way, but during recovery the adipostat becomes active once again.

Choosing a realistic body weight is usually only a problem for patients who have previously been at very low weights, as they may wish to remain or achieve low body weights which are difficult to maintain, unless the woman is preoccupied with food and dieting, which hinders progress to recovery. It is interesting that many patients who have been at high body weights often select as their desired weight one which is still above the normal range, for example, a BMI in the ranges 25–29. The woman should understand that she is not expected to maintain a constant weight, as fluctuations of 0.5–1.5 kg (1–3 lbs) are normal and are due to daily fluctuations in water balance and contents of the intestinal tract. Unless the woman is aware of this, she may respond to an increase of 0.5 kg (1.1 lbs) with panic, and this may precipitate an episode of binge-eating. On the other hand she may respond to a small loss of weight by thinking that she can eat more and this may start an episode of binge-eating. For these reasons a woman who has bulimia nervosa should stop weighing herself or at least avoid weighing herself more frequently than once a week, as this may precipitate feelings of panic, inadequacy, or failure.

A binge-eater has to learn to control her disordered eating behaviour before trying to reduce her weight, as any serious attempt at dieting will usually result in binge-eating episodes. This requires frequent discussions with her therapist, and often with a dietitian.

The object of these sessions is to help the woman learn to eat the appropriate amount of food required to maintain her weight and resist the urge to binge-eat. This is achieved by persuading her to eat balanced meals at regular intervals, at least three times a day, with occasional snacks. Some meals will include 'guilt' or 'binge' foods which are introduced, one at a time, to allow her to gain confidence that she can eat them without having an urge to binge-eat, or to gain excessive body weight. Dietary guidelines are discussed to help her introduce these foods into her diet. She is not allowed, for example, to buy 'guilt' foods in large quantities and may only eat these foods in company, at least initially. Nutritional and dietetic counselling is also provided, as many patients no longer know how much they can eat in order to maintain weight. When patients describe the amount of food they feel they can eat, they do not take account of their binge-eating. For example, many patients are convinced that if they eat more than 5040 kJ (1200 kcal) a day they will put on weight, and they claim that they have to keep themselves on a reducing diet when not binge-eating. A skilful dietitian can help a woman learn normal eating behaviour without increasing her need to focus on food and become more preoccupied with food, eating, and weight control. It may take some time for patients to have enough confidence to accept that when they cease binge-eating, self-induced vomiting, and purgation they will be able to eat more at meals without weight gain.

In-patient treatment may be necessary for some patients to feel safe and confident that they can learn normal eating behaviour and can cease inappropriate weight-losing behaviour.

Avoiding inappropriate weight-losing behaviour

Although many binge-eaters are aware that 'starvation diets', self-induced vomiting, and laxative and diuretic abuse are potentially dangerous, their knowledge is often inaccurate. Treatment of binge-eating includes discussion of the use the woman has made of weight-losing methods and her willingness to reduce their use. Many women who binge-eat are willing, at least initially, to try to change their behaviour, and are reassured when they learn about the effects which may occur. Most are unaware that they may gain weight temporarily when they cease the behaviour, as they retain fluid in their body. Most do not know that after ceasing to use the behaviour, constipation may persist for some time, as well as a feeling of abdominal fullness and cramps. As these women are preoccupied with body weight and abdominal fullness, such symptoms make them anxious, which may precipitate self-induced vomiting and purgation, starvation or binge-eating. It is often helpful for the woman to think of the symptoms as 'withdrawal symptoms' which she will have to suffer for a period of time. After ten days of avoiding the behaviours mentioned, most patients usually feel comfortable; and after three weeks they usually report feeling better than they ever have, especially with respect to fatigue. Unfortunately it takes most patients some time to have the confidence to stop their behaviour completely, because they fear a rapid weight increase and loss of control of eating. It is difficult for them to be able to feel that their binge-eating will lessen if this behaviour stops and in-patient treatment may be needed for some women to achieve this objective.

Recognition of negative (dysphoric) moods

Patients describe anxiety, tension, and unpleasant moods prior to binge-eating. In most, the negative mood is relieved during or after the binge. A theory has been advanced which seeks to explain why the binge relieves the negative mood (see page 52). The theory relies on the belief that the brain level of a hormone called serotonin is low in people who are irritable, depressed, or anxious, in other words, those who have a dysphoric mood. If such a person eats a carbohydrate-rich meal or binges on carbohydrate-rich foods, the level of a substance called tryptophan in her blood is raised. The higher blood level of tryptophan permits some of the tryptophan to cross from the blood into the brain where it stimulates the synthesis and release of serotonin. This raises the level of serotonin in the brain and relieves the dysphoric mood, making the woman feel relaxed and drowsy. However the relief only lasts for a time, after which the dysphoric mood returns, and is relieved by eating another carbohydrate-rich meal or a binge. Recognition by the patient of the association between unpleasant moods, especially anxiety, and relief from them by binge-eating assists her to find other more appropriate ways of coping with tension. Relaxation therapy can help, if only to enable patients to recognize their anxiety. Many patients find relaxation difficult at any time and almost impossible prior to a binge when they are most agitated and tense.

Antidepressant drugs in the treatment of bulimia nervosa

Several antidepressant drugs have been tried to discover if they would reduce the frequency of binge-eating. The evidence of these trials is that antidepressants have a limited benefit in the treatment of bulimia nervosa.

The antidepressant drugs which increase brain serotonin (such as tryptophan and selective serotonin re-uptake inhibitors (see page 00) do help some women with bulimia nervosa to reduce binge-eating. Recent well-conducted clinical trials using fluoxetine (Prozac) with over 500 patients have now been published, and show that compared with a placebo, 50 per cent of the patients who took fluoxetine had significant reductions in binge-eating and vomiting during the 16-week trial period compared with less than 20 per cent of women taking the placebo. However the drop-out rate was high and the duration of the trial short. Other studies confirm the short-term benefits of fluoxetine and confirm that the patients who responded were those who were not depressed as well as those who had symptoms of depression. More studies are needed to explore the usefulness of these drugs over longer periods of time.

As the frequency of binge-eating decreases, the woman can discuss her need to eat in the face of tension or stress. Once she understands herself a little better, she can reorganize her life-style to minimize eating due to tension or stress, for example, when examinations are approaching, by working more consistently without a last-minute cram or by studying in a place which does not have easy access to food; by learning to have confidence to ask questions of, or help from, lecturers and tutors rather than worrying about what she does not know; or by arranging activities so she does not spend all day feeling she should study and eating as an excuse not to start. Some women, particularly those with a long history of bulimia nervosa, will explain that they 'binge' only so that they can induce vomiting. They become 'addicted' to vomiting to reduce tension.

Case history: Pat

I still have binges now—but they are shorter, they cause me less remorse and guilt, and I consume less food during them than before. I simply can't fit the *volume* of food in I could before. I am fuller sooner. They also relieve my anxious feelings better. I have the binge and I feel relieved. I can even sit and watch television for the rest of the night without continuing to eat, because I am *satisfied*.

When I was caught up in it before, the night would dissolve into an endless foray in and out of the kitchen. I might stop for 1–2 hours (when absolutely full) but restart eating later. Now, I usually stop and that's it—no more. (Although not always—I still experience a few binges like before and feel sick in bed afterwards.)

If I want to, I can stop the binge before it starts, or even *at* a point during it. But I have to say to myself: 'Why are you doing this? What's the matter? What are you trying to say to yourself?' or 'What are you unhappy about?'

Often the answer comes easily—'I'm unhappy about Bill, I miss him' or 'I had a fight with Kevin and he boxed me into a corner again' or 'I'm hassled. There are too many things to do and I don't know if I can do them all in time' or 'My mother-in-law was here today and she annoys me. She seems to take over *our* house (even though I know she doesn't) and when she's here everything revolves around her' (she's a semi-invalid).

Sometimes I don't know why I'm bingeing (unlike before when I *never* knew why I was bingeing). And then I can't stop the binge.

Now the binges don't affect my weight that much. Firstly, they mean less food intake. Secondly, I can make up by eating sparingly the next day (and I usually am *not* hungry for a while). Thirdly, I can run or play squash to adjust my weight and enjoy the exercise.

How strange to feel 'satisfied' and happy with your life! It is the most superb feeling, to feel good about yourself!

I am pleased with my body and what it can do for me (in terms of sport or sex). It is not as skinny as I had wanted nor is it a model's figure. But it suits me and two men have lately confirmed that, saying things I would never have thought possible, like 'you have a little bottom' or 'I like your legs'.

I have treated myself to the luxury of new, fashionable, trendy clothes—a joy from the days when I dreaded trying on jeans because even size 14 (UK size 36, European size 42) never fitted me. In fact, many of the clothes from previous seasons look dowdy and very boring now—they represented a me who was afraid to show any of her body,

Case history: Pat (continued)

who wore discreet plain clothes so as not to 'show off' and who never looked sexy because a fat person had no *right* to be sexual.

I know my body attracts men. I can feel the 'vibrations' or I can feel them watching me sometimes. This confirms my feelings of self-confidence in myself but also perhaps suggests that the new-found sexuality is showing. I feel a 'complete' person—all the pieces are there fitting together correctly—including the sexual part of me—and I guess it shows.

Binges for me are also a way to relax. I always keep little activities to do around the house so I am 'busy' and occupied away from food. But if I am tired or don't want to do them, then sometimes I'm stuck. I want to unwind and food is a good way. It involves little mental effort, it calms the nervous feeling in my stomach, and it takes my mind away from work or troubles.

The recognition of precipitants

The patient and the therapist explore and discuss those factors, such as marital and family stress (which we have mentioned on page 196), loneliness, tenseness, and boredom, which have precipitated binge-eating in the past and currently. Recognition of precipitants to binge-eating assists patients to reorganize their lifestyle either to avoid these situations or to find other ways of coping at these times. It is interesting that as patients improve they recognize hunger as a precipitant but also explain that previously they had trouble recognizing accurate cues for hunger and satiation.

Encouragement of resistance behaviour

As was mentioned earlier, most binge-eaters have tried to resist binge-eating at some time or another. The methods they have used are many and various, and exploration of these with the therapist can give the patient insight into the problem. Some of the less-extreme behaviours can be used successfully at times by patients and can be included in treatment programmes. Reorganization of lifestyle so that patients are occupied at the times they are most likely to binge-eat is useful, for example, attending a gym on the way home from work and before dinner, or washing hair and playing computer games when at home at night. Patients need a number of these interests, as they tend to become less effective over time, and the patient must enjoy the chosen occupation. Sensible exercise can be promoted for most bulimia nervosa sufferers, but the exercise needs to be controlled as some patients are at risk of developing an exercise disorder (see page 117) which may replace or co-exist with the eating disorder. The chosen exercise regimen must be perceived by the woman as enjoyable. For example, if the patient hates jogging or bike-riding, there is no point in suggesting that she jogs or cycles. Taking up interests also helps patients to feel better about themselves and feel more like other people.

Treatment of the physical symptoms

Most bulimia patients require little medical treatment for their physical symptoms. When treatment is needed it is usually because the woman has developed a potassium or a vitamin deficiency because of 'starvation diets', or self-induced vomiting, or abuse of slimming tablets, laxatives, or diuretics. In a few cases, treatment is needed because of a suicide attempt.

The symptoms of physical discomfort described by patients during or after binge-eating are: swelling of hands and feet, abdominal fullness, fatigue, headache, nausea, and abdominal pain. The swelling of hands and feet appears to be associated with the amount of food eaten and this symptom may be used by patients to obtain prescriptions from doctors for diuretics. The presence of the other symptoms appears to be associated more with the presence or absence of induced vomiting.

Management of gynaecological problems

Many bulimia nervosa victims have disordered menstruation. Their menstrual periods either cease or occur only infrequently. Investigation and treatment of menstrual disturbances is rarely needed, as the menstrual pattern will return to normal once binge-eating, starvation, vomiting, excessive exercise, and abuse of laxatives and diuretics have ceased. However, if the woman is at low body weight and has not menstruated for some months, oral contraceptives may be prescribed, as these may stop her bones becoming brittle. In such patients the lack of menstruation is associated with the woman's low body weight. In most bulimia nervosa patients, lack of menstruation seems to be associated with the eating and the weight-losing methods rather than low body weight, as the woman's weight is in the normal range.

If the woman is sexually active, oral contraceptives will also prevent her from unexpectedly becoming pregnant, as pregnancy may occur occasionally even if the woman has not started menstruating again.

During the period of recovery from bulimia nervosa, many women need reassurance that they will not have become sterile as a result of their infrequent or absent ovulation and menstruation.

Family relationships, social, and other problems

Marriage

For the woman who marries when she has active bulimia nervosa, the chance that the marriage will break down is double that of other women, although this is not the case if she marries before she develops bulimia nervosa or after it has been cured.

Many bulimia nervosa patients have problems relating to their age and their lifestyle which they have been unable to discuss with others. When they feel confident in their therapist they are able to start talking about these problems. In adolescent women a struggle may be going on between the woman and her parents, over her independence and the parents' need for a dependent child. Other bulimia nervosa patients are ill at ease in social situations, have a low self-esteem, and are uncertain of the direction of their life. They may find it difficult to relate to others. These problems have been discussed in relation to women who have anorexia nervosa (page 180).

During treatment, women report changes in their binge-eating behaviour. Some women say that they no longer binge-eat, only overeat, while others say that the feelings associated with a binge still occur from time to time but the amount of food eaten is small and the frequency is reduced. These patients have a good chance of ceasing to have bulimia nervosa.

A few patients simply decide to stop fighting binge-eating. They buy and prepare food to binge upon each day. In other words they stop the out of control nature of eating during a binge by being prepared and knowing when they will overeat. These patients have a poor outcome, as their eating behaviour continues to interfere with their social life, relationships, and career.

Support groups for parents and partners are also important, particularly soon after the problem has been discovered or while the woman is being treated in hospital. It is reassuring for parents and partners to know that other people have a daughter or a partner who has similar problems and to be able to share and talk through their fears and hopes. They also need to feel that they can have a regular contact with the people who are helping their daughter or partner.

The response to treatment

The binges still occur but I would define them now as 'over-eating'. My weight has gone up 3 kg (6½ lbs) but it doesn't bother me. I don't weigh myself anymore, at least not often. I don't try to stick to a diet as it would just emphasize food once again (but I'm sure that I will always count calories in my mind—but only in hundreds). I feel happy and try to eat normally whenever possible.

A good response to treatment is that:

(1) the woman ceases to binge-eat;

(2) she ceases to use potentially dangerous methods of weight control, such as self-induced vomiting, purgative abuse, slimming tablet abuse, or diuretic abuse;

(3) her weight is stable;

Table 34. Binge-eater's needs

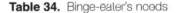

Be motivated to recover
To learn that dieting is unnecessary
To learn that most foods can be eaten in moderate quantities without a dramatic change in weight
To eat at least three meals a day
To discontinue vomiting and purging
To understand that urges to binge-eat certain foods may persist for many months
To meet with the therapist each week or every 2 weeks to plan for the next period
To stop dividing foods into 'good' and 'bad' foods
To learn to like herself

(4) she eats regular meals;

(5) she is able to interact with others of both sexes in social situations;

(6) her self-esteem is good and is not dependent on her body weight or shape.

Case history: Yvonne

It's good to feel 'normal' about eating and my weight now. I eat whatever I feel like, including cakes, an occasional chocolate, honey, bread, ice cream, rich savoury dishes like quiche or pies. I eat when I want to, but I have found that I enjoy food most when I *am* hungry and can sit, eat leisurely, and savour it. I have also found that my stomach will signal when it's full (although it's too easy to miss the signal at times) and I usually stop eating then. It's like regular people who eat when they're hungry and stop when they're full.

My appetite varies tremendously. Sometimes I will be hungry in the morning and eat breakfast, followed by something at 10.00 or 11.00 a.m., and then a bite at lunch. Other times, if I've had a big meal the previous night, a cup of tea takes me through till 12.00.

It amazes me how little food I need to satisfy my hunger at that moment. However, if I discover myself constantly in the kitchen searching for 'something' simply to put in my mouth, I realize I am bored or uptight and am seeking a pacifier. Then, I ask myself '*Exactly what* food appeals particularly?' Often the answer comes back 'Well, nothing really' or 'I don't know' and then (if I feel like it) I will say to myself 'You're not hungry really; you're just looking for a diversion' and go away to find something else to do.

My weight varies in cycles (this being deduced, not from the tyranny of the bathroom scales, but from the looseness of the clothes around my waist and bottom and the actual look of my stomach and lower chest—slight rolls being apparent at the heavier weight).

My weight does not worry me, nor do I try to control it by strict dieting. If I feel 'heavy', I will eat less food and drink less, watch carefully for that point of stomach fullness, and exercise more (running, dancing, gym classes, tennis).

There are cycles of heaviness when I feel heavy and have been overeating and even non-aggressive binges. It's nice to know the connection between weight and eating. I know I am eating more and I feel my weight going up—not like before when I always seemed 'fat' regardless of how much or how little I ate.

Case history: Yvonne (continued)

Then there are slim cycles when I feel slimmer, trimmer, and eat less (no sweets or dessert after dinner, no wine, no lunches out, no picking) but this just happens and I do not control it or feel guilty about eating less or more . . .

Recently, under much pressure of work and relationships, I started experiencing a 'knot' in my stomach, thinking it may be the start of an ulcer!

It immediately reminded me of my binge-days when I often had this knot and thought it was stomach (i.e. physiological) hunger. Then, I would eat to relieve the 'hunger'. Food soothed away the pain and did, in fact, make me feel 'better', no longer being plagued by a gnawing in the stomach. However, when I ate food or drank milk to relieve the knot, it relieved it temporarily but then left me in 5 minutes again feeling the same. It was a tension build-up and I learnt I could relieve it by deep breaths (trying to relax) or walking around and stretching. It went away after a couple of weeks.

It is important for the patient and her family to know what is the long-term outcome of bulimia nervosa. At present only two long-term studies over a period of 10 to 15 years, have been reported. One of them is our study of 50 consecutive patients (48 women and 2 men) diagnosed by Suzanne Abraham as having bulimia nervosa 10–15 years ago. Of the 48 women, one woman died from a drug overdose in the sixth year of follow-up, two women were lost to follow-up in the first five years, and two refused to participate in the 10 year follow-up, although they did take part in the five year follow-up. One of these woman still had symptoms of bulimia nervosa at five years and the other was cured.

The 10–15 year outcome study of the 43 remaining women showed that 50 per cent of them could be considered cured, 30 per cent still had features of an eating disorder and 20 per cent still suffered from bulimia nervosa, an 'eating disorder not otherwise specified', or the binge-eating disorder (see page 38). These women binge-ate less frequently and no longer induced vomiting or purging. It appears that for some women, there may be a continuum from bulimia nervosa, through the binge-eating disorder to recovery. None of the patients had anorexia nervosa.

The women who were considered cured had had no relapse for more than two years. However relapses within two years were common. They are usually precipitated by a life stress, such as an impending examination, a change of job, illness, marriage, divorce, abortion, or the birth of a dead or deformed baby. Additionally some women stop their bulimic behaviour only to replace it with an exercise disorder or alcohol dependence. This change does not constitute a cure, as relapses to bulimic behaviour may occur.

For all these reasons it is important for someone who has apparently recovered from bulimia nervosa to know that she can seek help from a therapist whom she trusts and with whom she feels comfortable should she feel that a relapse is occurring. She may also take the measures shown in Table 35.

The 30 per cent of women who had some features of, or behaviour associated with, an eating disorder 10–15 years after the first presentation, resembled 'normal' women who are concerned about their body shape and weight. These 'normal' women may have occasional episodes of binge-eating or of food restriction (as did some of our patients) but these episodes do not interfere with the woman's lifestyle. Such women have been identified in the community as 'restrained eaters'.

The other follow-up study which was conducted in Britain, also of 50 patients, reported similar findings.

Our study showed that a good outcome was more likely if the woman had suffered only from bulimia nervosa and had not had episodes of anorexia nervosa as well. She was more likely to recover fully if close members of her family had not been treated for psychiatric problems, such as depression, alcohol dependency, or anxiety disorders. This last finding suggests that genetic factors may contribute to the development of an eating disorder in some cases. Women were also more likely to recover if they had not been at high body weight before or during the disorder. The reason for this may be that these women are less able to accept that 'normal' eating behaviour will result in a stable body weight. An alternative explanation is that they have a discrepancy between their natural 'set point' body weight and their desired body weight.

In the short term, that is five years or less, the studies show that the sooner the patient first seeks treatment, the better the outcome.

Table 35. What to do if you feel that you may relapse

In the first two years after you have recovered from bulimia nervosa, you may at times have an urge to start binge-eating and purging once again. The urge usually is precipitated by a stressful situation.

What can you do to overcome the urge?
The best approach is to contact your therapist so that you can talk about your problem with her.

If you do not want to do this, here are some suggestions:
- think through your problem and try to find a way to overcome it, other than by binge-eating;

- try to keep yourself occupied;

- talk about your problem with someone you can trust—sharing a problem helps resolve it;

- work out, from a food diary if you want, when you have strong urges to binge-eat. At these times plan to meet friends, go for a walk, or do something unconnected with food;

- try to keep eating three meals a day, with an extra snack if you wish;

- do not weigh yourself; if you must, never more than once each week.

This finding emphasizes that a major problem to overcome is the delay of binge-eaters in presenting for treatment. In part, this results from the patient's secrecy about her eating behaviour. She may only accept that she has an eating problem after she has tried to stop, or has been placed in a situation where she has not been able to continue her eating behaviour without being discovered.

Summary of treatment of bulimia nervosa
Treat as out-patient or as in-patient

Help patient to:
- stop trying to lose weight
- stabilize weight in desirable range
- stop using weight-losing behaviour
- learn sensible, normal eating patterns, appropriate to lifestyle

- eat food at least 3 times a day
- decrease preoccupation with weight and food
↓

Throughout programme provide:
- supportive psychotherapy
- cognitive and behaviour therapy
- help for other perceived problems
- assistance to improve self-concept
↓

Once binge-eating and weight-losing behaviours have ceased, if the woman is still overweight and wishes to lose weight, sensible dieting may be attempted. However, dieting is usually not necessary as a slow persistent weight loss occurs over a period of months or years.
↓

Overall aim is to help patient to:
- live a normal life
- be able to cope with life

11
Obesity

My other good news is that my weight isn't such a worry any more. I am still overweight, but I certainly don't feel the grotesque elephant I used to feel. I'm 72 kg (159 lbs, 11 st 5 lbs) at the moment which is low for me, and I haven't put on any weight for about seven months. I'm not really dieting I guess . . . just eating pretty sensibly and that seems to be enough to keep my weight stable. I know it's a slow and black way to lose weight, but this way my eating doesn't dominate my thoughts so much. I really do hope to get down to about 63 kg (140 lbs, 10 st) by Christmas and at that weight I'd like to think I'll be slim and satisfied with myself.

Obesity occurs when, over a period of time, the net energy intake exceeds the net energy expenditure. The term net energy intake is necessary because it has been observed that when a person increases the amount of energy ingested an increase in energy output occurs, and the excess energy available for storage in the body is less than 100 per cent of that ingested. The excess energy is stored in two main places in the body. The first place is obvious when you look at an obese person, that is, the energy is stored in adipose tissue. Adipose tissue consists of about 80 per cent fat, 18 per cent water, and 2 per cent protein. 1 kg (2.2 lbs) of adipose tissue has an energy content of 30 000 kJ (7150 kcals). The second storage area for energy is called the 'glycogen-water pool'. Glycogen is a substance found in muscle, and each gramme of glycogen is bound to 3.5 g of water. The combination of glycogen and water makes the glycogen-water pool. The exact size of the glycogen-water pool is difficult to measure, but it is thought to weight between 3.5 kg (7½ lbs) in a non-obese person and up to 5.5 kg (12 lbs) in an obese person. One kilogramme of the pool contains about 4200 kJ (1000 kcals) of energy, which is released (together with 3.5 kg [7½ lbs] of water) when energy is required and none is provided by food or drink. Only when the glycogen-water pool is almost depleted of energy is adipose tissue burned up to release energy.

Defining obesity

The body mass index

Obesity is defined in several ways, one being when the Body Mass Index is 30 or more (see page 24). The level of 30 has been chosen because statistics from life assurance companies indicate that above that level a significant increase in morbidity and mortality occurs compared with lower BMI. The level is rather higher than that derived from life insurance 'desirable' or 'ideal' weight-for-height tables. These tables were obtained after one particular company, the Metropolitan Life Insurance Company, had analysed the height and weight data of a large number of men and women and had found that 'desirable' or 'ideal' weights fell within a range. By desirable, they meant that people within this range of weights were at the lowest risk of developing illness or dying prematurely. When the 'desirable' range is related to the BMI the boundaries of the range of 19 to 24.9 fit approximately. People whose weight range lies in the BMI range of 25 to 29.9 are overweight, unless they are heavily muscled men, in which case their weight can be considered to be in the normal range. If their BMI is 28 or more, they have a slightly increased risk of developing some chronic illnesses such as a musculoskeletal disorder, but no increased chance of dying compared with people whose weight is in the normal range. A BMI of 30 to 34.9 is designated as *mild obesity*, between 35 and 39.9 as *moderate obesity*, while a BMI of 40 or more gives rise to a diagnosis of *severe (morbid) obesity*.

People who are obese run an increased risk of dying from heart disease (although smoking and high blood fats are stronger indicators), or from diabetes. The more obese the person, the higher the health risk (see p. 254).

Waist measurements

Another way of estimating obesity is to measure your waist circumference with a tape measure. A man's waist measurement of 102 cm

or more and a woman's waist measurement of 88 cm or more indicates that you are obese or have a high waist to hip ratio indicating
central adiposity (we discuss this in the section 'Apples and pears'
on page 253).

If a man's waist measurement is 94 cm or more and a woman's is
80 cm or more, it is a good time to obtain advice so that you can
decide if you want to lose weight. The reason is that beyond this
measurement, particularly if you are male, the risk to your health is
increased.

How common is obesity in the community?

It is actually rather difficult to determine how many people in the
community are obese. The first problem is that many research teams
use different definitions for overweight and for obesity. Secondly,
some reports include overweight and obesity in a single category—for
example, a report from the USA in 1990 showed that 30 per cent of
adults aged 20–69 were overweight or obese. This has now increased
to more than 50 per cent.

All investigators agree that in Australia, Britain, and the USA
more people have been identified as being obese during the past 15
years and the trend is continuing. This has led some people to
describe obesity as an epidemic of the new century. In Britain, the
number of obese adult men rose from 7 per cent to 17 per cent and
obese women from 13 per cent to 18 per cent.

As far as we can establish, about 23 per cent of American men
aged 20–69 are obese, as are about 24 per cent of American women.
We have more accurate data for Australia. In 1995 a National Health
Survey found that 19 per cent of men and 18 per cent of women aged
20–69 were obese as defined by a BMI of 30 or more. The numbers are
very similar in Finland where the population is surveyed every 5 years.
In 1997, 48 per cent of men were overweight and 19 per cent obese,
while in women the proportions were 32 per cent and 19 per cent. In
Britain it is anticipated that 25 per cent of adult men and women will
be obese by the year 2005.

If a person's BMI is 40 or more, he or she is *severely (or morbidly)
obese*. The prevalence of severe obesity is much less than that of
obesity, probably affecting fewer than one per cent of obese people. A
rough estimate is that one in 1500 adults in Western developed countries is severely obese.

Obesity and age

The prevalence of obesity and overweight people in a community increases with age. Information from several developed countries shows that between 9 and 14 per cent of children aged 8–11 are overweight. The most worrying recent trend is the increase in obesity in young children, age 8 to 11 years, living in the United States of America. This increase in the last 15 years includes a number of severely obese children who are suffering the adult medical obesity problems such as high blood pressure and diabetes. Amongst teenagers aged 14–19, between 11 and 19 per cent are overweight and between 2 and 5 per cent are obese. If a girl is obese in early adolescence (between the ages of 11 and 15) she has one chance in three of being or becoming obese by the age of 35. However, teenaged obesity accounts for no more than 10 per cent of all cases of adult obesity. Most adult obesity results from a steady, inexorable weight gain from the 20s onwards.

In Western countries the prevalence of obesity peaks between the ages of 55 and 65, when about 28 per cent of men and women are obese (Fig. 16). People whose parents were less educated and who are less educated themselves are twice as likely to become obese in their late 30s compared with non-manual or professional workers. Among women, three groups are more likely to become obese: women of lower social classes, women who do not marry, and women who have three or more pregnancies. The ability to lose weight

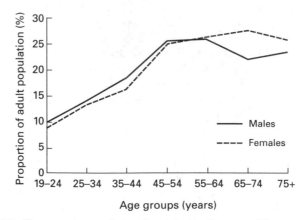

Fig. 16. The prevalence of obesity related to the age of the person.

following a pregnancy is currently of interest as there is preliminary evidence to suggest there maybe some genetic contribution to the ease of losing weight without exercise and dieting in the 12 months after the birth.

The increased prevalence of obesity with increasing age is in part due to the continuing ingestion of more energy each day than is expended; in part due to a reduction in the amount of energy the body needs for its basic functions as age advances; and in part due to a reduction in the amount of exercise taken as a person grows older.

In an affluent society where a wide variety of foods and drinks are available, and where advertising, particularly on television, plays a large part in food choices, most people tend to eat more than they need for their body functions and thus ingest spare energy. This extra energy is converted into fat. Among people whose weight is in the normal weight range (BMI 19 to 24.9), an average weight gain of 3 kg (6^1/$_2$ lbs) occurs between the ages of 25 and 45. The range of increase in weight usually lies between 2 and 7 kg (4^1/$_2$ and 15^1/$_2$ lbs) and rarely exceeds 10 kg (22 lbs). If the person has gained more than this amount there is a reason.

The psychological effects of being obese

In many cultures (for example Polynesia) a fat person is treated with respect and perceived as having a high social status. Within developing countries such as India, Africa, and South America obesity is becoming a problem among men and women as they become affluent, being overweight is seen by them as an indication of prosperity. In modern Western societies however obesity carries a social stigma. Obese children are seen as being stupid, dirty, lazy, smelly, and cheats. Fat adolescents are discriminated against by other students when at school, romantically, or when seeking a job. It has even been reported that health professionals perceive obese patients as less worthy of treating.

These attitudes naturally affect the emotional well-being of many fat people, which is one reason why many of them try to lose weight, often by adopting a fad diet. When the person loses weight, by what ever means, their mood improves, depressive episodes become fewer, and self-esteem rises. However if the weight loss is not maintained, the psychological symptoms may return. On the other hand, many overweight people try to ignore the prejudice and propagate the notion that 'fat is beautiful'.

As weight loss programmes are not particularly successful in the long term, many obese people will be satisfied if they lose some weight by eating a healthy diet, avoiding binge-eating and grazing, and exercising regularly. If they feel healthy they may choose to settle for being over-weight or mildly obese, in other words they have a 'reasonable weight' and should not feel guilty that they have not reduced their weight into the normal range. In fact there is evidence that if an obese person can achieve a 10 per cent reduction in weight, his or her health risks are reduced and the achievement is worthwhile.

The causes of obesity

Why do some people gain weight faster than normal as they grow older, tending to become severely obese in middle age? It is easier to start answering this question by listing factors which are no longer thought to be important in the case of most obese people, although one or more may operate in individuals:

- there is no increased absorption of food from the gut of obese individuals;
- there is no increase in thyroid deficiency among obese people;
- obese people do not appear to have greater 'addiction' for sweet foods containing more carbohydrate than thin people;
- the evidence that obese people choose a diet with a higher energy content than do thin people is not impressive. Further, in an experiment in which obese individuals were given two foods of similar appearance, one of which contained a high-energy content and the other a low-energy content, they were unable to detect any difference in the two foods;
- there is no conclusive evidence that obese people are less active than thin people.

When these hypotheses are excluded, the reasons why people become obese continue to be obscure.

A possible genetic factor

A genetic factor (or more probably several genetic factors) for some forms of adult obesity has been postulated. In 1994, a gene—the ob gene— was isolated. This gene induces the adipocytes (fat cells) to secrete a substance known as leptin. Leptin induces the brain to regulate food intake. Some obese people may be insensitive to the action of leptin and gain weight.

Other observations have added to the belief of a genetic factor in some cases of obesity—for example the study of twins. An American study reported in 1986 showed that the degree of fatness of nearly 2000 identical twins followed for 25 years was very close whilst that of 2000 fraternal twins was not so close. This suggested that heredity played a bigger part in obesity than environment, although both were important. Another way of determining if obesity is inherited is to see if body weight, and more particularly the BMI, of adopted children (when adults) related more closely to that of their biological parents than that of the adopting parents. A study made in Denmark in 1986 confirmed that the BMI of adopted children (when adults) related more closely to that of their biological parents, again suggesting that the tendency to obesity may be inherited. A third important study was also made in Denmark recently. The researchers were able to trace 57 people who had been adopted in childhood and to compare their weight and Body Mass Index with that of brothers or sisters who had not been adopted. The adoptees and their siblings when adult had very similar BMIs, in other words the fatter the adoptee the fatter his or her sibling was likely to be.

Additional support for the genetic factor in obesity comes from a French study. People who have a strong genetic reason for their obesity are likely to have been fat for most of their lives. Usually their fatness starts in infancy. The research team followed up fat infants for 20 years. They found that 40 per cent of the infants who were obese at the of one, were still obese as adults. Most of the infants did not increase their adiposity after the age of one until they were six years old. At that age a second phase of increasing fatness occurred among some of the children, and for those whose adiposity increased then, one in two children went on to become a fat adult.

The team also found that instead of putting on weight in spurts, as most children do, these children had a steady weight gain. In fact, over time their weight increased in a manner similar to their peers but at a higher level. They also found that the children were not slothful, being as active (or inactive) as other children in their age group. They were socially well-adjusted, because many of their relatives were fat and obesity was not perceived negatively. They accepted their body shape and image. If they tried to lose weight, they found it very difficult or impossible.

The conclusions that can be derived from these four studies are that a tendency to fatness is inherited, and this genetic factor may be as important in the development of obesity as behavioural factors which lead to overeating. What is not known is what percentage of fat people are overweight because of genetic factors.

How do genetic factors lead to obesity?

A genetic reason for obesity does not explain why fat people are fat. It has been suggested that what may happen is that a fatness gene or genes programme makes some people use the energy they absorb from food for their needs more efficiently than thin people. This means that people who will become, or who are, obese use less energy for any given activity, including their resting metabolism, than thin people and the excess of energy obtained from food intake is converted into fat and stored. It is important to note that for all but the most active people sedentary activities (which includes the body's resting metabolism) account for most of the daily energy expenditure. Recent studies show that obese people are genetically programmed to be more efficient in handling this proportion of their energy expenditure, although they use the same proportion of energy for exercise as lean people.

These findings receive additional support from research made by a group of British scientists. They found that healthy, sedentary obese men had inherited a lower proportion of a type of muscle fibre (slow muscle fibre) in their body than sedentary lean men. In their study, the men with a low proportion of slow muscle fibres burned less fat during work, in other words handled energy expenditure more efficiently, and consequently gained weight more readily.

Although attractive, this theory may not be correct. The development of a method of measuring energy expenditure using 'double-labelled water' and new instruments have permitted scientists to measure energy expenditure accurately in people living a normal life and not in the artificial environment of a laboratory. Using this technique, scientists in Britain have shown that a group of women who became fat during pregnancy, and remained fat after birth, had a higher resting metabolic rate (see page 257) than a group of lean women, and expended a quarter more energy (not less) each day than the lean women.

Is obesity due to a person having an increased number of adipose (fat) cells?

Another theory is based on the observation that an obese person has a larger number of fat cells in his or her body than a thin person. Until recently it was believed that fat cells only multiplied in the body until puberty. After puberty, if a person absorbed more energy from food than was expended by metabolic processes or by exercise, the excess energy was converted into fat and was stored in the existing fat cells which increased in size. It is now known that when faced with the challenge of fat to be stored at any age, the fat cells first increase in size and, when a critical size is reached, divide to form new fat cells. Once formed the fat cells never disappear. If a person continually eats more energy than she uses up, in every period that weight is gained an irreversible increase in the number of fat cells occurs, which in turn are able to store more energy in the form of fat, and the person becomes increasingly obese. It appears that obese people have bigger fat cells than lean people, and very obese people have more and bigger fat cells. If the theory is true, obesity should be prevented from childhood by establishing sensible eating habits so that the person avoids becoming obese. Once a person has become obese, particularly if severely obese, it is difficult for her to lose weight because of the large number of 'hungry' fat cells which 'demand' to be filled. In some way, messages reach her brain stimulating her to eat more. However, if the person has avoided becoming fat or is only slightly obese, fewer fat cells will have been produced and weight reduction is easier. Unfortunately, these descriptive observations, if true, do not help to identify what messages, biochemical or electrical, induce the person to adopt a disturbed eating habit.

Psychological reasons for obesity

The psychological reasons for obesity are not well understood. Psychologists have found that some people who feel that they are not appreciated, have lost their self-esteem, or are consistently dependent on others and always want to please them, binge-eat or 'graze' to overcome their negative feelings. If this behaviour continues over a long period, the person become obese. A problem with this theory is that many people who have a low self-esteem are not obese.

Another psychological reason contributing to obesity may be that subconsciously some fat people habitually underestimate the amount of food they eat. Support for this comes from a study by British researchers who asked nine fat and thirteen lean women to keep a record of the amount and type of food they ate over two periods of seven days. The researchers found that the fat women recorded eating less than the lean women. As the only explanation was that the fat women were eating more than they said they ate or they would not have been so fat, the scientists concluded that the fat women had underestimated their food intake and were unable to admit to themselves that their actual food intake was higher than they believed it to be. This belief has been confirmed in a study using the 'double-labelled water' technique. The researchers found that two-thirds of the people they studied, habitually underestimated the amount of food they are.

Additional support comes from a very careful study of 11 diet-resistant obese people made in 1992 in the USA. All of these people underestimated their food intake and overestimated the amount of exercise they took. This explains why some obese people fail to lose weight when on a low energy diet, but it does not explain how they become fat in the first place unless they underestimated their food intake from early life, or had a raised adipostat (set point).

It is known that many obese people snack between meals and indulge in 'picking' behaviour, eating chocolates, cakes, and sweets (foods which are rich in energy) at varying times during the day. They enjoy a few glasses of beer, or raid the refrigerator for soft drinks. They eat not because they are hungry but because they find eating pleasurable. They do not perceive the snack as food, and having eaten it, forget that they have eaten or drunk anything.

If these findings are correct, the occurrence of obesity in some families may be as much due to eating behaviours as to genetic factors. Fat parents may have fat children because the family enjoys food and are big eaters: food and eating are perceived as socially pleasurable and desirable. It is possible that these fat people are less easily satiated by food, in other words they feel 'full' more slowly. This could be the genetic reason for their obesity but unfortunately what makes a person feel 'full' after eating a particular amount of food is unknown, so it must remain a theory.

In Chapter 3 we gave some reasons why some adolescent women become overweight or obese. We suggested it was because they fail to reduce their energy intake after their growth spurt (and consequently their need for extra energy) has 'peaked' at about the age of 14. Women in families who enjoy eating are more likely to fail to reduce their food intake and become fat.

Some people who become obese do so for the same reasons as the overeaters but, as well, they tend to overeat or binge-eat when faced with a psychological or emotional problem. Their excessive eating may be precipitated by a disruption to their life or by an illness. They tend to be slothful, often dependent on others, and sensitive to criticism. They cope with stress, disappointment, a life-crisis, or depression by overeating. If overeating becomes a habit, because the pleasure of food blots out the pain of the problem, the person will gain weight inexorably. In both of these groups, habit and learned behaviour may be important in regulating food intake.

Summary for the possible reasons for obesity

In summary, the reasons why fat people become and remain fat are poorly understood, but over the years fat people must ingest more energy than they expend. For example, if a person are 1260 kJ (300 kcals) more energy each day than she expended, and if the net gain of this energy was 420 kJ (100 kcals) (after allowing the increased energy loss due to increased heat production), a net gain of 1533 kJ (365 kcals), which is equal to 4 kg (9 lbs) of fat, would occur each year. Recently there is increasing evidence, in men, that behavioural factors in eating control are important in the regulation of body weight.

Obesity, like many other human characteristics, is due in varying degrees in different people to a mix of genetic factors and behavioural factors. Heredity provides a tendency to obesity; eating behaviours either encourage or control that tendency. This means that learning to control eating behaviour is crucial if obesity is to be avoided.

Binge-eating among obese people

Recent studies have shown that 10–30 per cent of obese people engage frequently in binge-eating, and some have the binge-eating disorder or suffer from bulimia nervosa. The greater their weight the more likely are they to binge-eat. During a binge there may be considerable variation in the amount of food eaten. In most cases, obese binge-eaters, unlike bulimia nervosa sufferers, do not counter their binge-eating behaviour by vomiting or purging, and may or may not restrict their food intake between binge-eating episodes.

Obese binge-eaters tend to have a preoccupation with their shape and weight, but their control over their eating behaviour is poor. The management of obese binge-eaters is to combine cognitive-behavioural therapy with the other measures we will discuss later.

Childhood obesity

Obese children are disadvantaged children. From an early age obese children are seen as being lazy or as lacking self-control or as undesirable by adults and, more seriously, because of the greater psychological impact on the child, by their peers. They are mocked, laughed at, and sometimes castigated by lean people of all ages. In spite of being vulnerable to criticism most obese children manage to cope without becoming psychologically disturbed. This is fortunate because treatment of obesity in children is generally unsatisfactory. The surgical methods of weight reduction available for carefully selected adults (see page 280) are unjustified for children and probably dangerous. For these reasons, interventions to prevent excessive weight gain in children should be initiated earlier rather than later. However no action should be taken until the child is at least two to three years old, as young children need a high level of fat in their diet for their energy needs and to 'coat' (myelinize) their nerve fibres. Most programmes for obese children seek to reduce the weight gain rather than obtain a loss in weight. This is realistic as the latter approach usually fails. Weight-gain reduction is achieved by inducing the family and the child to change their food habits and to eat a diet in which the energy content has been reduced appropriately. As well as this, physical activity is emphasized. In a recent study in the United States the amount of television children watch was limited by the use of a novel digital device and with the support of their parents. During the time the television viewing hours were decreased the amount of weight the children gained was decreased. The results are thought to follow from the reduction in the amount of eating associated with watching television and an increase in exercise.

Care must be taken when dealing with obese children to avoid 'victim blaming'. It is wrong to suggest that the child is fat only because he or she eats too much, and that adherence to a strict diet will solve the problem. Childhood obesity may be due to a genetic disposition to obesity, cultural attitudes to feeding children, family eating behaviour, psychological factors, or a combination of these.

In the management of childhood obesity, if the family (and the child) makes a decision that weight loss is desirable, the health professionals involved should be supportive, empathetic, and enjoy working with children.

Apples and pears

Men and women deposit fat on their bodies in different places. When men become obese, most of the fat is stored in the tissues surrounding the gut and belly. In other words men become apple-shaped. Women, on the other hand, tend to store fat around their hips and buttocks, becoming pear-shaped.

The fat cells (adipocytes) in the tissues surrounding a man's gut and belly are large and metabolically active. Fat is released readily from them when a man diets and exercises. This means that the fat is more easily 'burned off' and the man loses weight. The type and distribution of fat in a man's body is characteristic of the fat in an animal's body. Animals put on fat in times of plenty to help them through times when food is not available.

The fat cells in the fatty tissues of a woman's hips and buttocks are smaller and less metabolically active. Fat stored in these cells is released less easily, even in conditions of starvation. This may be because of an evolutionary demand which permits the woman to have some energy stored should she become pregnant.

Recent investigations suggest that many of the health hazards of obesity relate more to the distribution of the fat than to the degree of obesity. Fat deposited around the waist appears to be more likely than fat on the hips or thighs to lead to health problems. This has led some experts to say that if you are a man and your waist measurement is more than 102 cm or if you are a woman and your waist measurement is more than 88 centimetres, you are in the higher risk health category.

Men and women tend to respond differently to their obesity. Women are more concerned about their body shape and weight (but not about muscle mass) than men, and are more likely to diet to try to reduce their weight. Unfortunately, they are also less likely to succeed in losing weight as easily as men. This is because:

- women may have a lower resting metabolic rate than men;
- and lose fat less readily even when they starve themselves;
- women burn up less fat for a given amount of exercise than men;
- women have a lower thermogenic effect following eating food.

Obesity as a health hazard

The fact that a proportion of the population is obese and a smaller proportion is morbidly obese would be of little consequence if obesity was harmless to health. Unfortunately it is not, as was shown recently by a study group of the British Medical Research Council who stated:

> We are unanimous in our belief that obesity is a hazard to health and a detriment to well-being. It is common enough to constitute one of the most important medical and public health problems of our time, whether we judge importance by a shorter expectation of life, increased morbidity, or cost to the community in terms of both money and anxiety.

The effect of obesity on health has been investigated by many researchers, and is shown in Fig. 17.

It can be seen that a severely obese person has a three-times greater chance of dying than a person of 'average' weight and, the more obese the person becomes, the greater is the mortality. Obese people tend to die young: obesity shortens a person's life.

In 1825 an obese man wrote a letter to his doctor:

> Sir, I have followed your prescription as if my life depended upon it, and I have ascertained that during this month I have lost 3 pounds or a little more. But in order to reach this result I have been obliged to do such violence to all my tastes and all my habits—in a word I have suffered so much—that while giving you my best thanks for your kind directions, I renounce the advantages of them and throw myself for the future entirely into the hands of Providence.

Many obese people would agree and would argue that the misery of keeping to a strict diet, which does violence to tastes and habits, is not worth it, although it reduces the chance of dying prematurely.

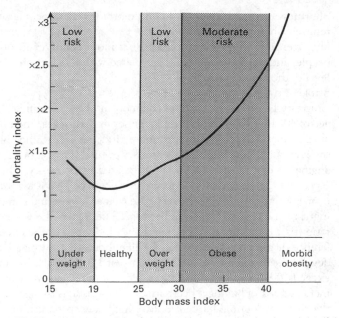

Fig. 17. The increasing risk of dying with increasing body weight. If the person's BMI is 37 he or she has twice the risk of dying compared with a person whose weight is in the normal BMI range. If his or her BMI is over 40 the risk is three times that of a person whose BMI is 20–25.

That is the person's choice; but obesity may not make life worth living. Obesity also increases a person's chance of becoming ill, and fat people are more likely to have a disabling disease than people of average weight. In other words obesity increases morbidity.

- Diabetes is five times more common among obese people, and is often cured when the person loses weight.
- Gall-bladder disease is more common in obese people and is more difficult to treat.
- Obese women have twice the risk of developing bowel or rectal cancer.
- Osteoarthritis, especially of hips, knees, and back, is more common in obese people; weight loss will not alter the disease, but is more effective than drugs in relieving the pain.

- Shortness of breath is usual among morbidly obese people: it is relieved when weight is lost.
- Hypertension (high blood pressure) is more common in obese people, and weight reduction is associated with a reduction in the level of the blood pressure.
- Stroke is twice as common in obese people.
- Coronary heart disease is more common in obese men under the age of 40; after that age the risk increases in both sexes, and obese women may have a disproportionate risk. Several studies have shown that 70 per cent of the 'coronary events' (heart attacks and angina) occurring in women are associated with obesity. This is especially so if the obesity is 'upper-body obesity'. This is identified by measuring the circumference of the woman's waist and comparing it to the circumference of her hips. The higher the waist-hip ratio (that is the circumference of the waist divided by the circumference of the hips) the greater the likelihood that a woman will develop heart disease in the next ten years. If the waist-hip ratio exceeds 0.9 in men and 0.85 in women, the person is at an increased risk of having a heart attack. The reason is thought to be that intra-abdominal fat cells release high concentrations of fatty acids into the blood going through the liver, which increases the level of fats in the blood.
- Menstrual irregularities (especially less frequent menstrual periods) increase as the weight increases, doubling in prevalence so that, among severely obese women, one in four has irregular or heavy periods. Obese women are also more likely to be infertile than women in the 'desirable' range of weight, mainly because frequently they fail to ovulate.

These rather negative findings may be converted to positive findings (Table 36). If an obese person loses weight so that her or his BMI falls to lie in the range of 19–24.9 or in the overweight range but less than a BMI of 28, she or he has less chance of developing diabetes, hypertension, a stroke, gall-bladder disease, and coronary heart disease than an obese person. Also, if the person has osteoarthritis it is likely to be less incapacitating. When an obese woman loses weight her menstrual periods become regular and, if infertile, she is more likely to become pregnant.

However it is important to be realistic and for the person not to aim at reaching a BMI which is below her 'set point', as the person

Table 36. The advantages of weight reduction

(1)	Reduction in blood pressure (both systolic and diastolic) (and consequently fewer strokes)
(2)	Improved cardiac function
(3)	Improved pulmonary ventilation
(4)	Reduction in pain from osteoarthritis and low-back pain
(5)	Improved circulation in legs with decrease in venous thrombosis
(6)	Reduction in fatigue: increase in energy
(7)	Increased self-esteem, increased social gregariousness, better 'body image'
(8)	Increased physical activity possible
(9)	Improved sexual relationships

may feel that he or she has failed if the unrealistically low BMI is not achieved.

The investigation of obesity

The medical and family history

The history should explore any reasons why the person is obese. Questions should be asked in a sensitive manner and the health professional should not make the obese person feel guilty or ashamed about being fat. Some people visit a health professional merely to be reassured that even though they are overweight or obese they are healthy and do not need to reduce their weight.

The history includes inquiring about any family history of obesity, looking for a possible hormonal cause, investigating any relationship or social problem, determining whether the person has any current medical condition (such as diabetes, osteoarthritis, or high blood pressure) which is causing concern, and finding out if he or she has previously attempted seriously to lose weight.

The history of the person's eating behaviour should be investigated as described in Chapter 6, and enquiry should be made to find out if the person binge-eats and has periods of strict dieting interspersed with binge-eating.

Other aspects that should be addressed in the medical history include alcohol consumption, smoking, and the use of illegal drugs. If the person is female, her menstrual and reproductive history is taken.

The questions outlined in Chapter 6 may prove useful in eliciting this information.

The psychological assessment

The aim of this assessment is to find out why the person has sought help. Most obese people have been overweight for months or years before seeking help. During this time over one-third have had frequent episodes of binge-eating. One obese person in five episodically binge-eats, compared to one in 20 in the overall community.

When the person seeks help, something has generally happened to precipitate her concern about being fat. It may be that she has been consistently teased about her appearance, or has been prodded to seek help by a person close to her, or that her health has worsened and she believes that obesity is the cause.

Her story should be listened to and her emotions, such as sadness, disappointment, or over-concern should be addressed at the same time as treatment is offered.

The physical examination

The physical examination is similar to that made when a person attends a doctor for an insurance examination, and includes an estimation of the blood pressure and an examination of the urine.

Laboratory tests

Laboratory tests have a limited place in the general physical examination according to British doctors, although American bariatric physicians disagree. Dr Garrow, in Britain, states that most of the tests often carried out, for example, X-rays of the skull (pituitary fossa), plasma insulin levels, glucose tolerance tests, secretion of cortisol and catecholamines, are of little value in evaluating obesity. On the other hand, Dr Bray in the United States, analyses blood samples for glucose, blood urea nitrogen, uric acid, alkaline phosphatase, total protein, serum glutamic oxalo-acetic transaminase, lactate dehydrogenase, bilirubin, thyroxine, triglyceride, and cholesterol. A sensible compromise would be for the patient's doctor to make selective biochemical and hormonal tests, explaining to the patient the reason for the tests, rather than ordering a battery of tests.

Following the history and general physical examination, several specific investigations may be required to determine the most appropriate treatment and the probable duration of time required for the person to achieve his desired weight, particularly if the person is severely or morbidly obese.

Assessment of the degree of obesity

Body composition

The body can be thought of being composed of two main compartments: fatty tissue and lean body mass. The fat compartment consists almost entirely of adipose tissue. The lean body mass consists of muscle, bone, non-bone tissue, and total body water. The total body water is the largest portion of the lean body mass. The body water occurs in all body cells (intracellular water) and the water which surrounds the cells and makes up a major part of the blood. It is possible to measure most of the compartments which make up the body either directly or indirectly.

Obese people have an increased amount of adipose tissue in their body and the greater the degree of obesity the larger is the adipose compartment. Thus, morbidly obese people have a large amount of adipose tissue, and their excess weight is mainly due to fat, but a few retain a large amount of water, which forms a significant component of their excess weight. It is important to differentiate the two types of people by determining their body composition. This can be done clinically and by using laboratory techniques. Both are required to fully establish body composition.

Why do overweight and obese people try to lose weight?

You might think that the potential and actual dangers of obesity to a person's health would be the main reason why so many people try to lose weight. This is not so, except in the case of some people who are moderately obese (BMI 35–39.9) and the few who are severely obese (BMI 40 or more). The reason may be that most of those who decide to lose weight are young or in early middle age, and they perceive the chance of developing a disabling disease as remote.

In the countries of Northern Europe, North America, and Australasia, most people, especially women, diet and exercise because they believe that by losing weight they will feel happier, look more attractive and in consequence, be healthier. The desire to lose weight even among those women whose weight is in the normal range, or in the lower range of overweight (BMI less than 28) is influenced by the pervasive messages of the media, as discussed in Chapter 1.

The majority of women who enter a diet and exercise programme only adhere to the programme for a relatively short period of time. After a diet-free interval they again embark on a diet, and so on. This pattern of weight control cycling ('yo-yo' dieting) is believed to lead in many cases to binge-eating. The theory is that periods of restrained eating—dieting—are replaced by periods of excessive eating, because of changes in the appetite (satiety) centre in the brain. See page 54 for a further discussion of binge-eating among obese patients.

Clinical estimates of obesity

The simplest method of determining the degree of obesity is to measure the Body Mass Index (see page 24). It is also useful to determine the proportion of body fat. This is inferred by making measurements of the thickness of a fold of skin at four sites on the body.

The following skin-fold thicknesses are measured by picking up a fold of skin and measuring its width with callipers (Fig. 18).

(1) *biceps skin-fold* over the front of upper arm midway between elbow and shoulder;

(2) *triceps skin-fold* over the back of upper arm midway between elbow and shoulder;

(3) *subscapular skin-fold* under lower tip of the shoulder blade;

(4) *suprailiac skin-fold* above the crest of hip bone.

The information obtained from the sum of the four skin-fold measurements is used to estimate the fat as a percentage of the body weight by referring to special tables constructed for each sex and age range. The results, when compared with the specific laboratory tests outlined in the next section, show that skin-fold measurement gives a close indication of the percentage of fat in the body.

Laboratory estimates of body composition and obesity

In obesity research, laboratory investigations are used to increase our knowledge about body composition and about obesity. One of the measurements of interest to scientists is the amount of fat a person has in her or his body. As we have just mentioned, this may be obtained by measuring skin folds which give a good approximation of body fat and are generally all that is wanted. However, a more exact estimation may be needed. This can be obtained by obtaining the person's body composition, including the proportion of adipose tissue, using a dual energy X-ray absorbiometer (a DEXA) machine. The woman lies on a couch and the whole procedure takes about 20 minutes. The method is safe, less than half the amount of radiation being released than occurs in a chest X-ray, it is non-invasive, relatively cheap, and gives accurate measurements. The DEXA enables scientists to measure the total body mineral density (as well as the bone density of regions such as the spine and the legs), the lean body mass, and the percentage of adipose tissue (fat) in the body. These additional measurements are important to middle-aged women, as a low bone density, for example, indicates that the woman is more likely to develop osteoporosis in later years, unless she takes action to prevent this happening. The DEXA machine has largely replaced the complicated method of measuring total body water which used to be the yard-stick.

Some research scientists want to measure the resting metabolic rate (RMR) of a person: that is, the amount of energy used for basal body functions. This is done by measuring the woman's total body

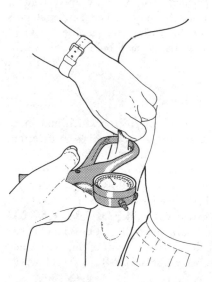

Fig. 18. Measuring skin-fold thickness with callipers.

potassium, by injecting an isotope into her blood and detecting its release using a spectrometer.

Individuals of the same sex, age, body composition, and body weight have different energy requirements for their resting, unconscious functions of breathing, body repair, heat control, intestinal activity, etc., and, in addition, they use energy with different degrees of efficiency for muscular activity. In practice, muscular activity is a less important factor than the RMR in determining a person's energy expenditure. Obese people generally have a higher RMR than lean people, but the energy used by obese individuals differs considerably. This will influence rate of weight loss if an obese person chooses to diet.

The management of obesity

Weight loss is not easy and those people who decide to try to lose weight can be helped by three complementary strategies. The first is to lose weight by eating less and by resisting the urge to eat. Treatment for this strategy seeks to help the person to keep to the chosen menu plan and to be motivated to continue to keep to the plan over a period of several months. It also means that she should be aware that she tends to underestimate how much she eats.

The second strategy is to persuade the person to take regular, enjoyable exercise in addition to the menu plan. The third strategy is to help the person make changes to her eating and exercise behaviour and lifestyle and discuss how these changes will help prevent weight gain in the future.

Exercise as a means of losing weight

Lack of exercise—sloth—is recognized as a factor which may make obesity worse or hinder weight loss. If someone takes in a certain amount of energy from food it is obvious that the more exercise that she takes each day, the less energy is left to convert into fat. Unfortunately, people have to be very active to use up excess energy (that is, excess to the body's basic needs) obtained from food. For example, a serving of breakfast cereal with milk provides about 700 kJ (167 Kcal), an orange 50 kJ (36 Kcal), and a slice of bread and butter or margarine about 800 kJ (191 Kcal). The amount of time you would have to exercise to use up this energy is shown in Table 37. However,

Table 37. Energy expenditure of certain physical activities

Activity	Average time (in minutes) required to burn off different amounts of energy		
	Energy burnt off		
	400 kJ	800 kJ	1200 kJ
Walking, golf (21 kJ per min)	19	36	57
Cycling, tennis, swimming (30 kJ per min)	13	26	40
Jogging, squash (42 kJ per min)	9	19	28

regular exercise, especially if taken after meals, may have a specific action in helping weight to be lost, although this seems to vary from person to person.

Although Table 37 shows the length of time an activity should be undertaken to achieve an equivalent loss of kilojoules, different exercise regimens have different benefits. Jogging, for example, puts stress on joints, which swimming does not. Swimming has the disadvantage that the body is supported by the water and less energy is burnt off. Exercise machines are expensive.

Probably the best, most efficient, and least damaging exercise is walking, but in choosing an exercise programme, the person should choose the one which most appeals to her or him.

The important factor is that you do the exercise regularly, for example, walking briskly for at least 30 minutes, at least three times a week. You should start gradually and increase the frequency and duration of the length of time spent exercising. It is also worthwhile remembering that activities such as house-work, walking to the shops, gardening, and playing golf are all activities which involve physical activity.

As an addition to eating wisely, exercise improves physical fitness and helps weight loss. It must be done regularly and exercise which is felt to be enjoyable by the person should be chosen.

Weight-reducing programmes

The reason that we prefer 'weight-reducing programme' to a weight-reducing 'diet' is that most diets fail. This is because the woman concentrates on the diet sheet and ignores the other issues which will enable her to lose weight. Many diets have been devised and many have failed to produce either the desired weight loss or permitted the person to maintain the new lower weight permanently. A few strictly controlled diets (such as the very low calorie diet VLCD which we mention on page 278) help very obese people to start losing weight, and are successful in the short term. But a person who wishes to keep her weight in the normal range, needs a weight-reducing *programme*. During the weight-reducing programme, the woman learns new eating behaviours, which are not seen as 'dieting' but rather as acquiring *normal eating behaviours* (see page 226) which will continue after she has lost the desired amount of weight.

Weight loss is a slow process, and the patient may become despondent about achieving it. The support, information, and encouragement offered by a group such as Weight Watchers or TOPS (Take off Pounds Sensibly), or a psychologist or a physician and a dietitian will enhance the patient's motivation, encourage her skills, and offer help in dealing with situations which may trigger the urge to eat excessively. It is also evident that the greater the patient's original weight the longer is the period required to enhance her motivation, and the greater the chance that she will abandon her attempts. In this situation, surgical intervention, in spite of its dangers, may be appropriate provided that the patient fully understands the implications of surgery and that the long-term 'success' rate has not been clearly defined.

Slow rather than rapid weight loss preferred

Before the patient embarks on a weight-reduction programme it is important for a physician to make sure that the weight loss is medically desirable and psychologically wise. It is even more important for the obese person to accept that an average loss of weight of 0.5–1.0 kg (1–2 lbs) is the maximum usually obtained after the first few weeks (when a weight loss of 2–4 kg [4–8 lbs] a week may occur) and the most appropriate programmes are designed to help the person achieve this small but steady loss of weight. But, as in the treatment of anorexia nervosa or bulimia, a weight-reducing programme alone is not enough; motivation to resist the urge to eat and to keep to the programme is essential.

It will be recalled that excess energy is stored in the body in adipose tissue and in the glycogen-water pool. If a person starves in order to lose weight, or at least considerably reduces her energy intake, she extracts energy from the stores in her body to meet the energy needs. The first source of energy comes from the glycogen-water pool. The size of the pool varies. In non-obese people it weights about 3.5 kg (7^1/$_2$ lbs). In obese people it weighs about 5.5 kg (12 lbs). It contains about 4000 kJ (1000 kcals) per kilogramme. When energy is released from the stores in the glycogen of the pool, water is also released. For every 1000 kcals of energy released, 3–4 kg (6^1/$_2$–8^1/$_2$ lbs) of water will be lost to the body in breathing, as sweat, or in urine. In the first weeks of a severe reducing diet, or of starvation, a quick weight loss may be expected as the energy in the glycogen-water pool is used up and a large quantity of water is lost to the body. However, the energy in the pool will be depleted within 1 to 4 weeks (when a weight loss of 3–6 kg [6^1/$_2$–13 lbs] will have occurred). After this time, any further weight loss has to come from 'burning-up' the adipose tissue to release energy. The second component of weight loss is a slow, steady loss. The amount lost weekly will depend on the restriction of the energy take, but rarely exceeds 0.5–1.0 kg (1–2 lbs) per week.

An obese person who wishes to achieve a weight reduction of 45 kg (99 lbs) has to lose the equivalent of 1 320 000 kJ (315 000 kcals), as each kilogramme of adipose tissue contains 29 300 kJ (7000 kcals). If she takes a diet supplying about 4620 kJ (1100 kcals) a day, which provides an energy deficit of about 4620 kJ (1100 kcals) loss of weight over her energy needs each day, she should achieve this in about 10 months, but the rate of weight loss will depend on her lean body mass and on her metabolic rate. The higher her metabolic rate, the quicker will her weight loss occur, so that the time taken varies and only a range of time can be given to the individual, unless research laboratory facilities are available to calculate her resting metabolic rate.

There is a further problem. When a person loses weight and stabilizes her weight at a lower level, her body reacts and 'resets' her metabolism at a lower level. This may mean that even if she continues to adhere to her menu programme and takes regular exercise, she may find it hard to maintain her lower weight and it slowly increases. The problem may be aggravated by her feeling constantly hungry and wishing to eat. It is thought that this may be the effect of an 'obesity gene' (see page 242) acting on a centre in the brain, the 'satiety' centre or adipostat, which somehow regulates the amount of fat in a person's body.

The consequence of this is that if an obese person tries to lose weight and fails, she may correctly say that she has kept to her weight-reducing programme. She should not be made to feel that she has failed. She needs support, not criticism.

Case history: Marjorie

It all started about 10 years ago, on my parents' 25th wedding anniversary, when my sister's husband deserted her. We were all living at home and we had endless family discussions, which became very emotional. And at the same time I became increasingly worried about the business ethics of my employers; they were crooked. These two things made me tense and angry all the time. To top it off my boyfriend had a bad accident and became very depressed so he needed my support. I felt that I was everybody's prop and couldn't escape.

I wasn't aware of it at first that my weight began to rise, until I found I needed a size 16 dress instead of a size 12. I tried to diet but the problems remained and food seemed to be the only way I could dull the pain. I got into the habit of looking in the mirror, being depressed at what I saw and eating some more so that I could cope. I dieted and began losing weight, and then I'd give it up and eat enormous amounts and gain weight once more.

My behaviour became destructive to me. I now knew I was using food as an escape from emotional pain and stress. I was really no different from an alcoholic, and I realized I wasn't going to conquer it alone but there was nowhere to go. I was on a roller coaster of eating and dieting and I couldn't get off. I didn't induce vomiting or take laxatives or anything like that. It wasn't as if I had thought of these things and rejected them—I hadn't even thought of them.

I knew I had an eating disorder. I wasn't in control; food was controlling me. I was a fat girl and I wanted to be thin, but I couldn't keep to a diet to become thin. I'm still a fat girl. I now weight 86 kg (140 lbs, 14 st). I wish I could get thinner.

The weight-reduction programme—three components

The weight-reduction programme has three components. These are: that the woman accepts a menu plan; learns new eating behaviours; and takes regular exercise. Exercise has been discussed on page 258.

The other two components of the programme will now be considered.

The menu plan

It is best to consult with a dietitian about a menu plan to ensure the menu is suitable for you, is nutritionally adequate and that you will be able to achieve. The principles of the menu plan of the programme are shown in Table 38. They meet several important criteria. The programme permits a wide variety of food choices, it is well-balanced nutritionally and it reduces the amount of energy ingested. It enables the person to eat varied, palatable meals so that she does not feel 'different' from family or friends.

Experience has shown that the weight loss in the first four weeks is crucial. At the end of this time three outcomes are possible. First, if the person has lost 4–8 kg (9–18 lbs) and says that she did not find it difficult to keep to the menu plan, future progress is likely to be satisfactory. Second, if the person says that, after four weeks, she has lost less than 3 kg (6^1/$_2$ lbs) and has found it increasingly difficult to keep to the menu plan, or says that she has kept rigidly to it and has lost less than 3 kg, the possible reasons for the poor weight loss should be investigated. The most likely cause is that the person's home or workplace environment is such that the temptation to eat snacks cannot be overcome. In this case cognitive therapy (see page 114) may help the person to keep to the weight-reducing programme. Third, the person may fail to lose significant weight in spite of having kept strictly to the programme. Such people require further investigation,

Table 38. The principles of the menu plan

1. It must supply *less* than the person's energy requirements.

2. It must provide all nutrient requirements except energy.

3. It must be acceptable to the person.

4. It must be sustained.

5. It must not impair health or well-being (e.g. low-fibre diets may cause constipation).

6. Its effectiveness will depend on the foods the person *refrains* from eating.

including in some cases an estimate of the person's resting metabolic rate, as described on pages 257–8.

If you choose the menu plan of the weight-reducing programme you have to make some decisions. The first is that you must reduce considerably the amount of fat you eat. This means that you only buy lean meat and trim off the extra fat. You can eat poultry, but not the skin because this is fatty. You should grill the meat rather than fry it. You may eat butter or margarine but you must spread it thinly. You should eat less cakes, chocolates, sauces, pastry, and many kinds of biscuit because these foods contain 'hidden' fats and 'hidden' sugars.

The considerable reduction of the quantity of fat you eat, together with regular exercise, are the most helpful ways in which you can reduce your weight and maintain the lower weight. You do not need to count calories.

The second decision is that you may also need to restrict the quantity of some *carbohydrate* foods which you eat. You may need to reduce the sugars added to cereals, tea, or coffee and avoid some sugar-rich foods such as sweets and candies. Diet spreads and jams may be useful in reducing energy intake. After talking with your dietitian you may also need to reduce the energy content of your drinks. In any addiction, withdrawal of your 'drug' may cause upsets. When you reduce the sugar you are having you may find that you crave to add it to your tea or coffee or to your breakfast cereal. You can deal with this craving for sugar in one of two ways. Which you choose will depend on your personality. The first way is to stop at once. You may use a sugar substitute in tea and coffee and on breakfast foods. You also avoid drinking large amounts of fruit drinks, including those which claim to have 'no added sugar', because they contain fructose which is in the fruit. The second way is to be more gentle with yourself. If you habitually add three spoons of sugar to your cup of tea, cut it down to two, and then after a few days to one. In other words, wean yourself gradually from your craving for sugar and sweet foods.

Third, you should cut back your intake of alcohol or, preferably, avoid drinking any alcohol. Although alcohol is not strictly a carbohydrate it provides energy in the same way. And many of us enjoy a drink! Again, you can be very firm with yourself and drink soda water with a slice of lemon and, if you wish, a dash of angostura bitters in place of your favourite drink. Or, if you are less strong, you can if you wish have half a pint (250 ml) of beer, or a nip (30 ml) of whisky, or a glass (125 ml) of a light wine a day. Each of these provides 25 g (a little under an ounce) equivalent of carbohydrate, or about 420 kJ (100 kcals) of energy. Diet mixes/sodas may be useful in reducing energy intake or you can add water or soda water which contain no energy.

The attraction of this sensible menu plan is that within certain limits you eat much the same foods as the rest of your family, and so you don't feel outcast or different.

It may well be that while you are on a menu plan you are invited out to a dinner party. You don't have to be embarrassed, or embarrass your hostess, by toying with your food and leaving most of it on the plate. If you just try to stick to your menu plan as closely as possible, be sensible, and enjoy yourself.

A menu plan, which is low in energy and in carbohydrate and rich in fibre, has many advantages. It is nutritious; it is relatively easy to understand and to follow; it doesn't make you feel a freak; it avoids gimmicks; you can stay on it for a long time, and, most important of all, it works! These criteria form the basis of a sensible diet for a sensible person.

Learning new eating behaviours

A menu, in itself, will not enable a person to lose weight, however carefully it is devised and however many dietary cook-books are made available. The person has to be motivated to keep to the plan and to understand it. Unless the person is motivated, she will find it easy to cheat—just a little! But lots of 'just a littles' equal a considerable amount of excess energy ingested. Motivation can be encouraged in several ways, and the woman requires to choose the way which she finds more appropriate for her.

Many people find that their motivation to lose weight is increased if the person can share her experiences with, and obtain support from, other people who are also trying to lose weight. The support needs to extend over a period of weeks or months during the period of weight reduction. Support is also needed when the person has achieved the lower weight, so that she does not regain weight swiftly or insidiously. Many obese women find it helpful if they join an organization such as Weight Watchers or TOPS.

Membership of the organization provides a stimulus to achieve a weight loss (by a system of rewards and demerits) and provides a form of group therapy. The value of such organizations is shown by a study made in Australia in which the weight loss of women attending a hospital-based obesity clinic was compared with that of women who joined Weight Watchers. The women who had joined Weight Watchers lost more weight each week and remained at the lower weight for longer than those women who attended the obesity clinic.

Motivation and information

Motivation and knowledge is also required because there is no magical, easy method of losing weight. It is fairly easy to lose 3–6 kg (6^1/$_2$–13 lbs) of weight quickly, but it is difficult to prevent the relentless return of that weight unless the person is sufficiently motivated to continue eating energy than is used up in daily living. Weight reduction is a slow process, but if a person is sufficiently motivated to keep to a diet providing 2100–4200 kJ (500–1000 kcals) less than is needed each day, stored fat will be burned up at a rate of about 0.5–1.0 kg (1–2 lbs) a week. The time that it takes to lose weight may be better understood if we consider as examples two women, both aged 42 and both 162 cm (5 ft 4 ins) in height. Both work outside the home, part-time. One woman weighs 60 kg and the other 100 kg. The first woman wants to lose weight. The body composition of the two women is shown in Table 39.

Table 39. The body composition of two women

	Woman A		Woman B	
Age	42		42	
Height	162 cm		162 cm	
Weight	60 kg		100 kg	
BMI	22.8		38.0	
Body composition	*kg*	*%*	*kg*	*%*
Lean body mass				
Water	30.0	50	43	43
Protein	9.0	15	12	12
Minerals	2.4	4	4	4
Glycogen	0.6	1	1	1
Adipose tissue	18.0	30	40	40

It can be seen from this table that the second woman has 40 kg of adipose tissue in her body, 22 kg more than the first woman. If she follows the menu plan of the weight-reducing programme she will ingest 5050 kJ (1200 kcals) of energy a day. As her body needs 9240 kJ (2200 kcals) of energy for its functions, she will have an energy deficit each day of 4200 kJ (1000 kcals). Fat has an energy content of 37 kJ per gram but about 10 per cent of it is needed for metabolic process in converting the fat to energy, so that about 33 kJ will be available to reduce the energy deficit. As the daily deficit is 4200 kJ, she will burn off between 115 and 130 g of fat each day (the actual quantity depends on a number of factors). That works out at about three-quarters of a kilogram (1½ lbs) a week. So that to lose the desired 22 kg she will have to continue her diet for six months to achieve her desired weight.

Another example is given in Beryl's story, which also shows the difficulty of keeping to the 5040 kJ daily intake of energy unless the woman is motivated.

Case history: Beryl

Beryl is an obese, middle-aged woman, whose height is 1.60 m (5 ft 3 in) and who weighs 72 kg (159 lbs, 11 st 5 lbs). Her BMI is 28, so she is overweight. In fact she is about 17 kg (37 lbs, 2 st 9 lbs) more than she would like to be, and most of this excess is due to fat she has made and stored over the years when she has eaten more energy in the form of food than she has used up. Beryl has read articles and is worried about being too fat. She would like to get back to a weight of 55 kg (121 lbs, 8 st 9 lbs). Each day she probably expends about 8400 kJ (2000 kcals) of energy to meet the demands of her body and her work in the house. If she could manage to eat only 4200 kJ (1000 kcals) a day, it would take 125 days—over four months—before she exhausted her stored energy by burning up the fat she had laid down over the years. She talks about losing weight with her doctor, but thinks that she would find it difficult to stick to a menu plan providing only 4200 kJ (1000 kcals) a day, and chooses a menu plan which provides 6300 kJ (1500 kcals) a day. On this diet, if she sticks to it exactly, she would burn up 2100 kJ (500 kcal) of stored energy each day and it would take her 250 days—over eight months—for her weight to fall to the ideal! Beryl has a real problem, for it is stupid to pretend that it is easy to lose 17 kg (37 lbs, 2 st 9 lbs) of weight and it is unlikely, whatever diet she decides upon, that she will manage to do it in less than eight months.

> *Case history: Beryl*
> As well as this, previously obese people who have managed to reduce their weight by dieting regain weight very quickly, compared with untreated fat people, if they start over-eating again. For this reason, Beryl will have to exert very great will-power to achieve her weight loss and to keep to her lower weight.

The motivation to keep to the chosen reducing diet is increased if the person is aware that even when she keeps to her diet rigorously, her weight may fluctuate within 1–2 kg (2–4 lbs). For this reason she should avoid weighing herself more frequently than once a week.

It is also important that the diet chosen permits the person to enjoy a social life. It is pointless and counterproductive to be a thinning, anti-social, crotchety recluse—it is better to be fat and enjoy life. Becoming thin should not be made a punishment, nor should an obese person be filled with guilt as well as fat. A well planned weight-reducing programme recommended in this book (and other sensible programmes) enables a person to eat with the family and to socialize with friends.

Other behavioural strategies

There are other behavioural changes which a person who is trying to lose weight may choose to adopt. However, if any of them makes the person think continually about food it may hinder rather than help her keep to her programme. This applies especially to obese people who binge-eat. For this reason, care should be taken to choose those changes which can be adopted comfortably. They can be listed as follows.

• When on the programme take more exercise—if you enjoy it. Don't exercise and hate it. You may compensate for your dislike by over-eating. It is helpful if you go for a walk, or do something active, after a meal. There is evidence that this helps you lose weight rather more quickly than if you slump down in front of the television set as soon as you have finished eating. This is because exercise induces heat production and energy loss.

• Don't go on a 'crash diet' which provides less than 2100 kJ (500 kcals) a day unless you are under careful medical supervision. Initially these diets produce a rapid weight loss, but after a while you will find you cannot keep to the diet, and when you stop you usually over-eat. If you persist for over a month eating a crash diet and semi-starving yourself, your body reacts by reducing your basal metabolic rate by up to 40 per cent, so that you burn up less energy than if you eat a sensible weight-reducing diet providing between 4200 and 5000 kJ (1000–1200 kcals).

Crash diets and crazy diets do not really help, despite what the magazines and your friends say. For a short while they seem to succeed. The reason is that most of the weight lost is water (from the glycogen-water pool) and not fat. Sooner rather than later, you find that you cannot keep to the crash diet and you overeat. Your weight increases and you become discouraged!

There are two reasons for this. The first is that it is very difficult to keep to an uninteresting diet for long enough for it to be effective, except in the very short term. The second reason is a physiological one. When eating a very low kilojoule diet, the dieter's resting metabolic rate drops rapidly and may decline by 20 per cent within two weeks. This means that although she loses weight fairly rapidly for the first two weeks, after that time the weight refuses to melt away. Also her body adapts to the strict diet by secreting more of an enzyme, lipoprotein lipase, which regulates how much fat is stored in the fat cells. This makes her body more efficient at storing fat, which is precisely what she doesn't want.

To avoid these problems someone who intends to use a weight-reducing programme may be helped if she follows some simple rules.

• Choose a menu plan which is nutritious, and which is sufficiently varied and tasty to enable you to stick to it without getting bored or frustrated. As far as weight loss is concerned you should focus on reducing your energy intake, rather than counting calories. You should eat both complex carbohydrates and a certain amount of protein. Your menu plan should also contain sufficient vitamins, minerals, and dietary fibre ('roughage') to keep you in good health. But make each meal attractive to look at, pleasant to smell, and good to taste, so that you learn to enjoy what you ear.

• If you limit the dietary fibre in your food you may become constipated and be at an increased risk of developing cancer of the large bowel, coronary heart disease, and haemorrhoids. The remedy is easy: eat wholemeal bread or one or more of the fibre-rich foods mentioned earlier.

• Don't gorge by eating only one large meal a day. You will lose weight more quickly if you eat several small meals spread out over the day—and you will feel normal if you do this. Do not miss breakfast and do not eat your last meal late at night. The reason for eating several small meals rather than a single large meal is that smaller meals eaten at shorter intervals induce a greater production of body heat (the 'thermogenic' effect of food), which is then dissipated into the surrounding air. Body heat is produced by using energy, and that is what you are trying to do—to use more energy than you ingest.

• Try to eat sitting at a table and use utensils when you eat. Try not to distract yourself by watching TV, reading, or walking about when you eat, as you will eat more. Sitting down to eat also helps to train you not to eat when out walking past shops selling food and 'take-away' outlets, or when shopping. Eat your meals at approximately the same time each day. This has the psychological effect of helping you to control your feelings of hunger at times other than meal-times.

• When you have a meal, eat slowly. When you have put food in your mouth do not add any more until your mouth is empty. If it helps, put down your knife, fork, or spoon while your mouth has food in it. And chew your food slowly so that you learn to taste and smell the food to the fullest extent. Psychologists believe that eating slowly and chewing meticulously teaches you to be satisfied with less food and to enjoy the smaller quantity more. Additional dietary fibre will also help you to achieve this objective.

• Before you start eating, decide how much of which food you are going to put on your plate, and do not add more. Once you start eating it is too easy to say to yourself, 'I'll just have a little more.' You must not. 'Littles' add up to a lot and you will not control your eating. It often helps if you put your food on a smaller plate, so that the plate looks fuller! This will help you make do with less.

• As soon as you feel full, stop eating, no matter how much is still on your plate. Indeed, it may help you always to leave some food on your plate, and so break the habit of continuing to eat until all the food on your plate has gone, whether you need it or not.

• Once you feel full or finish your meal, leave the table (if you can do so without offending anybody). Staying at the table where there is food may break your resolve not to eat any more.

• Don't keep packets of sweets, biscuits, chocolate, chips, or nuts in the house or office. If you get bored or unhappy you will be tempted to have a nibble. If they are not there you can resist the

Table 40. The principles of a weight-reduction regimen

- Eat less
- Aim for a weight loss of about 2 kg a week for the first 2 or 3 weeks, then 0.5–1.0 kg a week
- Eat three meals a day, choosing from a variety of foods in the four main food groups: cereals and bread; vegetables and fruit; meat, poultry, and fish; dairy products
- Remember that your eating habits need changing in addition to reducing your energy intake
- Increase the amount of exercise you take each day. Exercise increases weight loss, and may cause metabolic changes which enhance further weight loss

temptation. If they are, you will be able to resist everything except the temptation.

- Only go shopping for food when you have eaten. If you do your own shopping, or shop for the family, you may be tempted when you see the delicious-looking foods in the shops. You can resist the temptation to buy and eat these foods if you do three simple things. First, only go shopping after you have eaten. People react less to the sight of food when they are not hungry. Second, make out a list of foods you really need before you go shopping. Stick to the list. Do not be tempted by other foods. Third, when possible, only buy foods which need more preparation than just opening the container. This will reduce the risk that you will 'just open a tin or a packet for a little snack'.
- Don't be 'conned' into choosing a complicated or expensive diet. You will not keep to it. Diets which insist that you only eat certain food on certain days, and other foods only at certain times of the day, should be avoided. They are rubbish. Choose a menu which is no more expensive than your usual food. If you do not, someone will complain and you will become discouraged and start eating more than your menu plan.

Drugs in the management of obesity

The role of drugs in the management of obesity is currently seen as an adjunct to the core treatments of behaviour therapy aimed at modifying eating-related activities, exercise to increase energy expenditure, and menu plans to lower energy intake.

Although the use of anorectic drugs and of thyroid hormone has been enthusiastically promoted in the treatment of obesity, their value is limited. All have been shown to have unwanted side effects.

Anorectic drugs reduce hunger or increase a feeling of fullness (satiety), but most obese people do not eat because of hunger. Nevertheless, carefully designed studies have shown that patients taking a low energy diet and anorectic medications lose more weight than those on a diet alone, but the effect diminishes or is reversed after about 12 weeks. And when the anorectic drug is stopped, weight is rapidly gained. The place of anorectic drugs in the treatment of obesity is limited, but they may be appropriate if the person's obesity poses a substantial health risk and for those who have to lose weight rapidly, for example, prior to surgery. Used in conjunction with diet, exercise, and supportive psychotherapy they help some patients come to terms with the need to lose weight over a long period, by giving them a 'prop' which helps to improve their morale. However, a study of the opinions of 1362 patients about the use of anorectic drugs showed that most preferred diet alone to diet and anorectic drugs. A minority of patients feel that anorectic drugs help. Anorectic drugs may achieve at least some of their effect by suggestion rather than by a direct action on the 'satiety' centre in the brain. This is suggested by an investigation which demonstrated that inert injections given to a group of patients produced a greater weight loss than that achieved by most active anti-obesity drugs.

Dexfenfluramine

An exception may be a drug, dexfenfluramine which is thought to increase the secretion of the brain hormone, serotonin (see page 54), and to prevent its uptake by the tissues, so that its levels in the brain increase. Serotonin appears to play a significant role in the control of the appetite. If the level of serotonin can be raised, the desire for food is reduced and the person may become relaxed and drowsy. If the level of serotonin is lowered, the person may become irritable or anxious and hungry, especially for carbohydrate-rich snacks. Studies using the drug show that dexfenfluramine increases the level of serotonin in the brain and reduces the person's 'snacking' and 'picking' behaviour, as well as reducing the appetite. Most of the weight loss occurs in the first 3 to

6 months, some weight may be lost in the second 6 months but there is no weight loss if the drug is taken for more than 12 months. In a multi-centre study of nearly 800 people (mainly women), half of whom were eating a restricted diet and took dexfenfluramine and the other half who just ate the restricted diet and were given a placebo pill, it was found that at the end of one year the mean weight loss of the group taking dexfenfluramine was 4 kg more than the people taking the placebo, and 30 per cent of them lost more than 10 kg compared with 16 per cent of the people who took the placebo.

When dexfenfluramine is discontinued weight is regained and unfortunately, the gain is more rapid in those people who lost greater amounts of body weight. Dexfenfluramine and a similar drug fenfluramine have been withdrawn from the market because of possible serious adverse effects. Each of these medications when taken in combination with another drug called phentermine, caused lesions in the valves of the heart resulting in an increase in the blood pressure of the lungs. It is not known if dexfenfluramine when taken alone can cause pulmonary hypertension. There have not been any cases reported.

Sibutramine

Sibutramine is a new drug that alters serotonin and noradrenaline reuptake in the brain. It is as effective as dexfenfluramine in inducing weight loss and is thought to have less adverse side effects. As with other drugs of this nature the symptoms of dry mouth, constipation, agitation, and insomnia may be a nuisance. This drug should only be taken with medical supervision and may not be suitable for all obese people, particularly those with blood pressure problems. This is the first drug of this kind to be used in the treatment of obesity and the long-term effects of taking this drug are unknown at this time.

Because of this, sibutramine, like other anorectic drugs, should only be tried if non-drug measures have proved ineffective. It seems to be particularly useful among people who have large appetites, binge-eat, or are nibblers or grazers.

Orlistat

Orlistat is a new medication that decreases the amount of fat you absorb from the gut. To enable the fat you eat to be absorbed by the body it must first be broken down into fatty acids and glycerol by the lipase enzyme in the small intestine (see page 282). If you eat a meal containing fat and are taking a lipase inhibitor such as orlistat the fat is not broken down and you pass fatty and oily stools. In fact eating a fatty meal may not be very pleasant as it can result in a lot of flatulence, smelly and fatty diarrhoea, urgency, and sometimes incontinence. Because of these unpleasant side effects people learn to reduce the amount of fat they eat and even learn to avoid the 'hidden fats' that are in the food we eat. In this way lipase inhibitors reduce energy intake and change people's eating behaviour and food selection.

Like all drugs associated with weight loss they must be taken under medical supervision. Because vitamins A and D are absorbed into our body dissolved in fat a few people may become deficient in these essential vitamins.

Fluoxetine, sertraline

These drugs selectively block the reuptake of serotonin (SSRIs) and are used in the treatment of depression. The first of these drugs was fluoxetine which is better known as Prozac. They do not stimulate serotonin release and do not have the adverse effects of dexfenfluramine when taken in combination with other drugs.

At lower doses, particularly in people who are depressed, these agents may allow the person to become more organized and compliant with lifestyle changes that promote the desired energy intake and output. At higher doses these medications increase satiety and promote weight loss. Recent studies indicate that the weight loss is modest, occurs in the first few months of taking the drug, and is not maintained. Both fluoxetine and sertraline lose their effectiveness as weight loss drugs with continued administration. It is not known why these agents lose their effectiveness and are no better than placebo (fake tablets) after 12 months. Other anti-obesity drugs continue to exert long-term anti-obesity effects and weight is not regained until the medication is ceased.

These agents are recommended as the antidepressant of choice for depressed patients who are obese. They may also have a short-term role in the management of binge-eating of some obese people and sufferers of obsessive-compulsive disorder.

Thyroid extract

Although thyroid extract is still popular among some doctors for the treatment of obesity, there is little evidence that it is of any value. The use of thyroid extract is based on the belief that people who are morbidly obese lack thyroid hormone. The inference from this belief is that thyroid tablets will reduce weight reduction. Thyroid tablets (available in two forms: thyroxine and triiodothyronine) increase the metabolic rate to some extent in people who have normal thyroid function, but the dose of the thyroid hormone required to produce any significant weight loss causes toxic symptoms in most cases. As well, the weight loss is mainly of lean tissue, not fat. In a careful study of the value of thyroxine in the treatment of obesity, no significant benefit was found over diet alone. Unless the obese person is hypothyroid, thyroid hormones should not be prescribed to increase weight loss.

Smoking

A number of people complain that when they stop smoking tobacco, because they have been advised that smoking increases their risk of heart attack and lung cancer, they put on weight. There is evidence that most people who stop smoking gain a small amount of weight (2 kg over a few years) and one person in ten (particularly if he or she is aged less than 55 and smokes more than 15 cigarettes a day) puts on more than 10 kg over a ten-year period. If the person is overweight and trying to lose weight this may be a deterrent. However, if the person reduces her or his energy intake still further for a few weeks, and increases their activity the problem usually ceases.

Summary of medical treatment for mild or moderate obesity

Clearly, if dietary measures and supportive psychotherapy enable the obese person to lose weight and maintain the body weight at the desirable level, surgical operations to help achieve weight reduction are unnecessary. It seems however that although almost any obese person can lose weight, few can keep it off. Many reports showing that a particular method was successful are methodologically unsound and have too short a follow-up. It has been demonstrated that most people who achieve an initial weight loss fail to maintain the lower weight for longer than 6 to 12 months. If the study terminates before 12 months, an inaccurate success rate will be reported. In longer-term studies made over 20 years ago, it was noted that few participants lost as much as 20 kg (44 lbs) and most who did regained weight shortly after treatment ended. A decade later, a large study in Britain showed that between 10 and 40 per cent of participants had lost some weight by the end of the first year of treatment, but fewer than 10 per cent maintained the weight loss for a period of years.

Modern approaches to the problem are first, to achieve realistic weight loss, and second, to maintain the lower weight by reinforcing the resolve of the person through periodic intervention in the form of supportive psychotherapy. These methods promise a more successful outcome. For example, a study of over 700 women who had reduced their weight over an average period of 30 weeks using the Weight Watchers programme, and who continued to attend group meetings periodically showed that 15 months after the weight loss had been achieved, only 30 per cent weighed more than 10 per cent above their 'desirable' weight.

An obese patient will only achieve and maintain weight reduction if she is motivated, persistent, and prepared to alter her lifestyle. If she is not prepared to fulfil these requirements, there is little point in persisting with a weight-reducing programme. The psychological assessment of an obese patient is an important diagnostic investigation. Many physicians believe that a full psychological evaluation by a clinical psychologist is necessary, but, from our discussions with our colleagues, and in our own experience, an assessment based on the questions asked in Chapter 6 is usually sufficient. However, if the assessment suggests that the habitual over-eating or binge-eating is associated with an underlying psychological problem, such as boredom, anger, depression, or 'stress', a clinical psychologist or a psychiatrist may help the person to cope with the problem and so cease to over-eat or binge-eat. Some obese patients find it helpful to keep a daily diary of all the food they eat during a week, noting where they were at the time, what they were doing, how they felt, and why they ate the food at that particular time (Food and mood diary shown in Chapter 7). The therapist is shown the diary and they discuss how the patient can change her eating behaviour. Many of the therapies mentioned in the treatments of the other eating disorders, including cognitive and behaviour therapies, are being used to help some obese patients.

Severe (morbid) obesity

The greater the degree of obesity, the harder it is for the person to lose weight permanently. Unless her health is so bad that a more drastic approach is necessary, the management of severe (morbid) obesity is first to try the medical and behavioural methods which have been described on pages 265–75. If these fail to effect a considerable weight loss, more stringent diets may be offered, particularly if the person is highly motivated to lose weight. These severe diets should only be attempted under strict medical supervision and with helpful support from a health professional who has experience in treating obesity. The alternative is to offer a surgical method.

The medical and behavioural methods include accepting a very strict diet such as the very low calorie diet (VLCD). The surgical procedures currently recommended are gastric stapling or laparoscopic banding, and in a few cases, gastric bypass. We will mention some other methods which have now been discarded because numbers of people who have had the procedures of jejuno-ileal bypass, and gastric balloon are in the community. Suction lipectomy (liposuction) used for cosmetic purposes, rather than weight reduction will also be discussed, as some obese women who have lost weight continue to be worried about the size and shape of their abdomen and thighs.

The milk diet

The need for a person to be motivated to keep to a diet which achieves a rapid weight loss over a relatively short period of time has led some British physicians to develop a diet which is easy to follow although extremely monotonous. The milk diet, as its name implies, consists of 1800 ml (3 pints) of whole cow's milk or a low-fat milk with supplementary iron, vitamins and, when necessary, an inert bulk laxative such as bran. The diet provides 4900 kJ (1170 kcals) of energy and 59 g of protein. Those who use it claim that the milk diet has several advantages over other diets. These are (1) it is cheap; (2) no weighing of foods or making food choices is necessary; (3) the diet is not complicated or troublesome to prepare. The obvious disadvantage of the milk diet is its monotony and that it inhibits the patient's social life, as she is often unwilling to go to social functions where a variety of food is available. A more important criticism is that the milk diet does not help to alter the eating behaviour of obese people. The diet can only be used for a short period of time for the reasons given. When the person returns to a more varied diet, she has not learned new eating habits and may rapidly revert to the previous patterns.

In spite of these constraints, the milk diet may be of value to some obese people, at least during the initial weeks of dieting. Once some weight loss has been achieved, the person should transfer to the weight-reducing programme, which provides a more varied, palatable diet, and produces a slow but steady weight loss.

The very low calorie diet (VLCD)

An alternative to the milk diet, the very low calorie diet (also known as the liquid diet, the Cambridge diet, or the 'protein sparing modified fast') may be tried. The diet is designed to provide no more than 42 kJ (10 kcals) per kilogram of the person's desirable body weight range (see page 24 to make the calculation). If you choose to start on the VLCD you must have a careful medical check-up before you enter the programme, and remain under medical supervision during the time you eat the VLCD because some people have died whilst on this very restrictive diet.

The diet provides 45–100 grams of protein, and is provided as a liquid formula. The diet also provides between 30 and 45 grams of carbohydrate and recommended levels of minerals, vitamins, electrolytes, and fatty acids to maintain health. In addition, dietary fibre is added. It is marketed under several trade names. The liquid is swallowed three to five times a day. The VLCD must be accompanied by increased physical activity.

The VLCD has a place in the treatment of very obese people who are not prepared to lose weight slowly, or who fail to lose weight using the weight-reducing programme, and who wish to try this method of weight reduction rather than having surgery.

The VLCD produces a loss of between 1.5 and 3.5 kilogrammes a week, but only one-third of people are able to keep to it for more than two months. A few very motivated people who are prepared to be under regular medical supervision continue for longer. Unfortunately after stopping the VLCD, even if they continue with a moderately low energy diet, most of them will regain much of the lost weight.

As with the milk diet, the VLCD may be used as an initial method for very obese people to lose weight, provided that it is followed by the weight-reducing programme and perhaps the addition of a drug (see p. 276) which seems to help in weight reduction. Preliminary studies using this strategy have shown that continued weight loss of 0.5 to 1.0 kg a week is achieved over the next 40 weeks.

However, there are several problems with the VLCD. The dieter loses protein from the blood and skin and the mass of the heart is reduced. A parallel reduction in the metabolic rate occurs which tends to reduce the effectiveness of the diet unless an exercise programme is also undertaken. Recent studies show that the VLCD should not be continued for more than 10–12 weeks as there is an increased risk that the person will develop gallstones. For all these reasons the VLCD diet which provides less than 3400 kJ (800 kcals) a day has limited value in the treatment of severe obesity, except in the short term.

Jaw-wiring

Those patients who fail to lose a significant amount of weight in spite of keeping to a 4200–5040 kJ (1000–1200 kcals) diet over a period of weeks or months, or who have an adverse social environment, may choose to have a surgical procedure which may protect them from eating more than their allowance. One such procedure is jaw-wiring. The molar teeth are wired, permitting the jaws to open only about half an inch (1.5 cm) (Fig. 19). This reduces the ability of the person to eat food, unless she removes the wire, homogenizes the food, or 'stuffs' food through the teeth. The person who has had her jaws wired is able to talk easily, but it will be obvious to her friends and relations that her mouth is relatively rigid when she speaks.

Before the molar teeth are wired, the patient has to agree (1) to attend her doctor at four-week intervals for evaluation; (2) to keep the jaws wired until the weight loss is such that no further medical

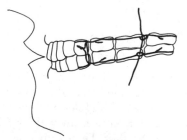

Fig. 19. The technique of jaw-wiring.

reason for weight loss persists; and (3) to continue dieting when the wires are removed. The reason for the last condition is that binge-eating is likely to occur after removal of the wires with consequent rapid weight gain.

Jaw-wiring is relatively painless, although some discomfort may be felt in the 24 hours after the procedure. This occurs from spasm of the jaw muscles, from bruising of the gums, or from toothache due to the sideways force on the teeth. Pain killers or sedatives may be required. A few patients develop ulceration of the inside of the cheek or the tongue from movement of the ends of the wires in the first few days after its application. This is easily corrected.

The jaws should not be wired for more than nine months as periodontal problems increase after this time. During the period the jaws are wired, the patient should be seen regularly by a dentist.

It may have become clear from this description that the purpose of jaw-wiring is similar to that of admission to hospital in anorexia nervosa. It is to control the person's eating and other weight-related behaviour until she has learned and can accept a new pattern of eating. From this it follows that although the procedure of jaw-wiring is simple, and physical complications are few, psychological problems may occur. The knowledge that the mouth cannot be opened may cause the person to feel a 'prisoner of her weight', and be attended by depression, or by a lack of ability to relate to her partner or family, particularly during the initial weeks after jaw-wiring. To cope with problems during this period, the patient needs moral and physical support from her partner and/or her family, and may be helped further with supportive psychotherapy.

As a steady, relentless weight gain seems inevitable after the wires have been removed, psychotherapy during this period may be helpful, but some people with morbid obesity may instead choose a major surgical operation to enable them to alter their disordered eating behaviour.

Major surgical procedures for the treatment of morbid obesity

The majority of people with morbid obesity will lose weight on a strict low energy diet. Many find it difficult to maintain their lower weight once the psychological support they received during weight loss is withdrawn, and within four to eight months many will have regained 50 per cent more of the weight they lost. These rather discouraging results induced physicians interested in treating obesity to review the physiology of digestion and to talk with their surgical colleagues.

The physiology of digestion (Fig. 20)

The primary function of the digestive tract is to provide the body with a continual supply of water, electrolytes, and nutrients. This is

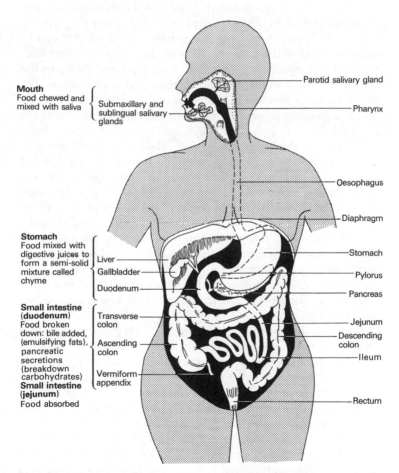

Mouth
Food chewed and mixed with saliva
{ Submaxillary and sublingual salivary glands

Parotid salivary gland

Pharynx

Oesophagus

Diaphragm

Stomach
Food mixed with digestive juices to form a semi-solid mixture called chyme
{ Liver
Gallbladder
Duodenum

Stomach

Pylorus

Pancreas

Small intestine (duodenum)
Food broken down: bile added, (emulsifying fats), pancreatic secretions (breakdown carbohydrates)
Small intestine (jejunum)
Food absorbed
{ Transverse colon
Ascending colon
Vermiform appendix

Jejunum

Descending colon

Ileum

Rectum

Fig. 20. The intestinal tract.

achieved by the movement of the food through the oesophagus, stomach, and intestines; by the secretion of digestive juices; and by the absorption of the digested foods, water, and electrolytes from the intestines.

The movement and mixing of foods occurs because slowly moving peristaltic waves of contractions pass regularly along the alimentary tract in response to its distension by food or water. These contractions squeeze the food onwards, mixing it at the same time.

In the mouth, food is masticated and mixed with saliva. It is then swallowed and passes through the oesophagus to enter the stomach. The stomach can store large quantities of food until it can be accommodated in the intestine. During its period in the stomach the food is mixed with gastric digestive juices and dilute hydro-chloric acid to form a semi-fluid mixture and is partially broken down. As space becomes available in the intestines, the mixture, called chyme, is moved from the stomach by peristaltic waves of contractions.

Most of the absorption of food takes place in the small intestine, where the chyme is acted on by secretions from the pancreas and by intestinal digestive juices. Carbohydrates are further broken down by the pancreatic secretions, and are absorbed, mainly in the jejunum. Fats are emulsified by the action of bile salts and digested by secretions from the pancreas and intestines to form free fatty acids, monoglycerides, and glycerol. In this state they are absorbed by the intestines, and the greater the distension of the intestines, the greater is the absorption. Protein is further broken down in the intestines into its constituent amino acids and absorbed. It is clear from these observations that most of the absorption of food takes place in the small intestine.

Understanding of these physiological concepts led to the idea that if most of the jejunum was bypassed by cutting it near its junction with the duodenum and anastomosing the cut end to the lower part of the ileum, the patient would be able to eat what she liked but would lose weight because the food would be neither digested nor absorbed. A second idea, which was developed somewhat later, as the complications following jejuno-ileal bypass surgery became apparent, was to reduce the size of the stomach. It was argued that if the size of the stomach was reduced by two-thirds, or more, the patient would be prevented from eating large meals because a feeling of fullness (or satiety) would rapidly come over her when she ate.

The effect of jejuno-ileal bypass (and similar operations) is to reduce considerably the amount of food absorbed from the gut, no matter how much food the patient eats. The principle of gastric reduction or partitioning is to increase the patient's reluctance to eat because she feels 'full' after eating a small amount of food. As it is the quantity of food which produces the feeling of satiation, an unmotivated person can cheat by eating or drinking small amounts of energy-dense liquids or food, most of which is absorbed. If a patient who has had gastric reduction does not cheat, this procedure (and jejuno-ileal bypass) will reduce considerably the amount of energy absorbed, and her weight will decrease steadily to reach her 'desirable' weight range after 6–15 months. It is also expected that the limited amount of food eaten, or energy absorbed, will enable the person to maintain her desired weight, once she had achieved it, and her weight will not increase.

The available operations have considerable disadvantages and some dangers. They should only be suggested to patients who are given full information about the surgical procedure and its effect and who have been carefully selected. The process of selection often involves a careful psychological evaluation to exclude severe emotional problems and to establish that the individual is properly motivated. The operations should not be seen as a 'quick fix' for gross obesity. They should only be offered by a team of doctors who manage obesity and who can provide the necessary follow-up.

Jejuno-ileal bypass

This operation was first introduced over 40 years ago, and in the 1970s became popular, particularly in the USA. As mentioned, the concept behind the operation was that if the duodenum and most of the jejunum were bypassed, foods (particularly fats) would not be absorbed. Heralded as very successful (as have been other operations for the treatment of obesity), experience showed that it had serious side-effects. The fat which was not absorbed remained in the bowel and prevented the absorption of the fat-soluble vitamins A and D. The breakdown products of fat in the bowel formed insoluble soaps

(a) (b)

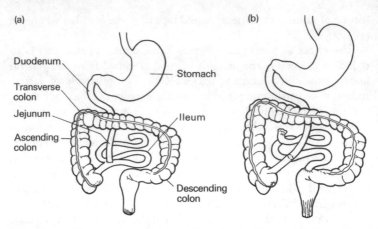

Fig. 21. (a) The end-to-side jejuno-ileal shunt of Payne; (b) the end-to-end jejuno-ileal shunt of Scott.

with calcium and magnesium, which increased the retention of water in the bowel leading to diarrhoea and to steatorrhoea. The frequency of bowel movements, and the chemical nature of the faeces, caused inflammation of the rectum in about one-third to one-half of patients, and led to an increased incidence of haemorrhoids. In the normal gut, calcium is bound to oxalate, but after jejuno-ileal bypass the oxalate becomes free and may be absorbed, leading to oxalate stones in the kidneys. Further, as other high energy substances in the diet, particularly carbohydrate, are also poorly absorbed, they are fermented by the bacteria in the gut leading to bloating and the formation of gas which is expelled either by belching or as flatus.

The long-term complications of jejuno-ileal bypass have been shown to be so severe, with a death rate of about 25 per cent in the five to ten years after surgery, and so common (Table 41) that a committee of experts developed and published a consensus statement in the *Journal of the American Medical Association* in 1981. The Consensus Statement said bluntly: 'In a current assessment of obesity management, one is compelled to reject jejuno-ileal bypass as a metabolically and physiologically unsafe procedure.'

Table 41. Complications and undesirable side-effects after jejuno-ileal bypass surgery

	Per cent of patients developing complications
Wound complications	15–25
Severe metabolic (mineral) disturbances	20–30
Ano-rectal pain/discomfort	35–50
Haemorrhoids	14–20
Severe (offensive) diarrhoea	15–20
Bloating, wind, flatus	10–15
Arthritis	8–12
Kidney stones	8–12
Gallstones	3–7
Psychiatric problems	6–10
Liver failure	3–5
Death	0.5–4
Re-operation required	10–20

Gastric bypass, gastric reduction, and lap-banding

Gastric bypass and gastric reduction as methods of reducing energy intake were less popular then jejuno-ileal bypass as earlier

Case history: Ken
I often sit and think back, was it worth all the problems I have been through.

It all started in 1969 when I asked for a new uniform as I was too fat for the old one, and I was told that I would have to lose weight, because there was not a wardsman's uniform in any larger size than what I already had.

So the next step was to see the staff doctor for a referral to a physician, who suggested that I attend a psychiatrist for hypnosis. I talked to my wife about this, and she suggested that I see a dietitian rather than a psychiatrist.

Case history: Ken (continued)

I did this but had no will-power to stick to a diet, because the slightest upset would make me eat and eat. So eventually I went along to the psychiatrist. But after a couple of visits, I was not too impressed and decided to go and try something else.

My physician was involved with jejuno-ileal bypass operation to lose weight and thought this might be the answer to my problems, but I should first try dieting.

He weighed me in at 130 kg (287 lbs, 20½ st; BMI 43) and took pulse, blood pressure and temperature readings and all the normal things, and then asked the questions about my past. I explained that at a young age I was not overweight; it was in my mid-teens that the weight started to build up. I took his advice and tried different diets but could not stick to them, and then I had a nasty experience.

I was walking up the hallway of my house and collapsed, I was taken to the hospital and the doctor there said that I had had a blood pressure attack, and that either I took the weight off within 6 months or I would have 6 months to live. At that stage I was 140 kg (309 lbs, 22 st 1 lb; BMI 46). I went on a 2100 kJ; (500 kcal) a day diet, and I was taking Duramine M40 tablets. I was also going to a doctor every second day and having female hormone injections, called chorionic gonadotrophin, which he said would guarantee I would lose weight.

In 5 months I lost 57 kg (126 lbs, 9 st). I kept this off for four years until late 1973, and then with my wife expecting our youngest son, and I was in threat of being retrenched from my job, I put all the weight back on again in 7 months, up again to 109 kg (240 lbs, 17 st 2 lbs; BMI 36).

After I had explained all this to my doctor, he told me about the operation in detail. He explained that the surgeon would bypass the small intestine leaving about 50 cm (20 in) but the remainder of the intestine would stay inside me.

Then he proceeded to tell me the side-effects such as diarrhoea, which would mean opening my bowels about five times a day, and that I might have wind pains and also a strict diet to stick to.

This sounded too good to be true; it was like waving a lollipop in front of a baby. So I agreed to the operation, and things went into action.

A date was arranged, and I went into hospital ten days before the operation was due to be performed. I underwent a lot of tests, such as: one day they would make me go without food, and the next day they would take core samples of fatty tissues from my buttocks. Then the

Case history: Ken (continued)

next day they would give me really fatty foods such as milk-shakes made of cream and radioactive fatty oil or something like that, and the next day the core tests would be done again.

Then came the operation. About 4 hours later I was back in bed, my wife was there and so were my doctors. I was, of course, very dopey.

In the next few days I went through a lot of pain, I was suffering a lot of cramps and wind pains, I also had a lot of vomiting, and as a result I was only allowed to drink a litre of fluid per day. Then the diarrhoea started, and after about 5 days the nurses sat me on the side of the bed, walked out and left me there. Five minutes later the bed tipped up, and I ended up on the floor wrapped around tubes and things, I could not move until they came back to help me. A doctor came to examine me to see if there was any damage done, and it was discovered that I had busted a tension stitch.

For the next 13 weeks I had a lot of diet and blood problems which were treated in various ways. I was released from hospital when these things were thought to be sorted out.

I was at home for about 3 weeks and was opening my bowels about 20 times a day, and I was very weak. My wife was suffering because of this, and was run off her feet with looking after me and running after the three children, as I could not do anything for her or myself.

I went back to see the physician and he had blood tests done and it was found that I had a low blood potassium. This was treated by admitting me to hospital and using a drip.

About 3 months after that, I was suffering a lot of abdominal pain, so I went back to him and he said I had an incisional hernia. I was admitted to hospital again and I had it repaired. I watched the operation as I had an epidural block, because I had such a bad reaction to anaesthetics.

Both of these problems (blood and hernia) repeated themselves; the hernia twice and different sorts of blood problems repeated themselves on numerous occasions, and were treated the same way, by admission to hospital. It seemed never-ending the weeks in hospital away from my wife and kids over a period of about four years.

I then started to go to a new family doctor, and after a period of time he discovered that I had a magnesium deficiency, so this was also treated. I went back again to the physician, and he noticed that I had a lot of muscle wastage on my left side, and I had practically no strength and was extremely weak. He said it was congenital, but my father said that I was a normal child. It was proved later that I had spinal nerve

Case history: Ken (continued)

damage. I have a lot of muscle wastage on my left side and sometimes my leg collapses from under me. This happened on one occasion and I fell and broke my right hip, which mean another operation to put a pin and plate in my hip; this was removed in September of this year 1982, 3 years after it happened.

From the constant diarrhoea, I have had about five fissure operations on my back passage; this happens about every 12 to 18 months.

All this has caused me to be off work for, so far, 8 years, and as far as I can see, there is no end to it all.

My weight now fluctuates between 76 and 79 kg (168 and 174 lbs, 12–12^1/$_2$ st; BMI 25–6). In the mornings I have a pretty normal flat tummy, but as the day goes on I blow up in the tummy like a balloon; as a result of this I have to have two sets of clothes, one set for the morning and another set for the afternoon to night time.

I have a blood test once a month and two injections once a month as well as a vitamin B$_{12}$ injection and a vitamin K injection. If I happen to be a few days overdue for these injections my muscles ache and I become pale and weak.

The operation has been successful as far as my losing weight is concerned, but if I had my way again, I would try something else as the emotional strain on myself and my family has left a lot of scars.

researchers found that the loss of weight was less. The initial suggestion was to reduce the size of the stomach by cutting it and to anastomize its upper portion with the jejunum (Fig. 24). In recent years this operation has been replaced by vertical gastric stapling (Fig. 25) which effectively reduces the size of the stomach, 'partitioning' it. A small aperture is left between the upper portion (the volume of which is made about 50 ml), and the lower larger portion. The size of the aperture is maintained by using a 'hemstich' of unabsorbable material. The size of the aperture appears to be crucial to the long-term success of the operation. The newest option is the placement of an adjustable gastric band called a lap-band. The lap-band consists of a solid silicone ring which is placed around the stomach about one centimeter below the junction between the oesophagus and the stomach. The band has an inflatable tube on the inside that is connected by a tube to a reservoir that is placed just under the skin. The inflatable tube attached to the lap-band, the tube and the reservoir are filled with saline. Removing or

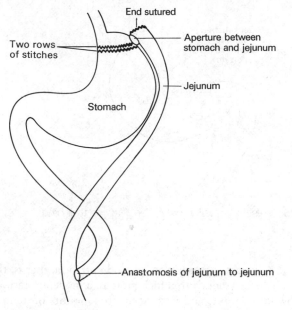

Fig. 24. Gastric bypass.

injecting saline into the reservoir can alter the tightness of the band
around the stomach. The band is positioned laparoscopically (key-
hole surgery), the stay in hospital is only 2 to 3 days and there are
few early surgical complications. It can be reassuring for people considering surgery for their obesity to know that the operation is
reversible and the stomach will return to its normal shape if the
band is removed. The tightness of the band can be released when
required, for example, during pregnancy. The effect of gastric
'partitioning' and lap-banding is that the person feels 'full' and
uncomfortable after eating a small amount of food, because the
small pouch is stretched and messages are sent to the 'satiety centre'
in the brain. Unless the patient eats slowly and keeps the amount
small, the pouch will fill and additional food will remain in the
oesophagus, leading to heartburn or vomiting. As both are uncomfortable, as is the feeling of 'fullness', the patient learns to reduce
her food intake and consequently loses weight.

Before an operation the person requires counselling and education in nutrition, as she will have to adopt to new eating behaviour.

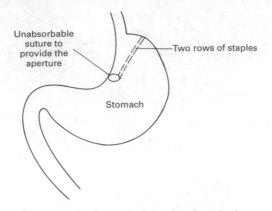

Fig. 25. Gastric reduction by vertical stapling (banding).

She will be taught the essentials of good nutrition, that is, the need to eat a balanced diet, with a high protein, a moderate carbohydrate and low-fat content, and with adequate amounts of dietary fibre, minerals, and vitamins; the patient is also taught how to cope with a greatly diminished gastric reservoir, the need to chew the food slowly and thoroughly, and the consequences which will occur (mainly vomiting) if she does not.

Gastric bypass and gastric stapling may also be followed by complications. Gallstones occur as frequently after gastric bypass as after jejuno-ileal bypass, vitamin deficiencies are frequent, and a few patients develop a stomach ulcer. Gastric stapling seems to be followed by fewer side-effects, particularly the metabolic upsets, than gastric bypass, but the follow-up period is short.

Gastric stapling must still be considered a potentially dangerous operation. The staples may separate, leading to leakage in the first days to a week after operation; the size of the pouch may increase, as may the opening between the upper and lower pouches. These changes enable a person to eat more without feeling satiated, or vomiting, and as soon as she can eat more she does, with the result that her weight increases. The lap-band is also not trouble free. The stomach can prolapse through the band, the band can erode into the stomach, the tube next to the reservoir can rupture and gallstones can develop. Removal and successful replacement of the band can be done for patients with prolapse or erosion problems.

There is no doubt that gastric stapling (or gastric bypass) will result in an average weight loss of 50 to 70% of excess weight over several years and is still 50% after 5 to 14 years. The success rate appears excellent but some patients do gain weight again. Following lap-banding patients lose weight rapidly over the first 12 months and more slowly during the second year, about 50 to 60 per cent of excess weight is lost which corresponds to a drop in BMI of 45 to 32. No further decrease in weight occurs after two years in studies that have continued for five years.

Gastric balloons

The complications that may follow gastric partitioning led some surgeons to develop a new approach to reducing the size of the stomach, by introducing a balloon into it. When the balloon (called a 'gastric bubble') was blown up, it had the effect of reducing the effective size of the stomach (as far as the processing of food was concerned) to a degree similar to that obtained by gastric stapling. Initially the 'gastric bubble' was hailed as a major breakthrough (shades of the jejunoileal bypass!) but soon severe side-effects were being reported. It was found that some patients developed gastric ulcers and some stomach perforations occurred. Occasionally the bubble collapsed spontaneously in the stomach requiring major surgery, or it led to intestinal blockage.

Unfortunately the early experience with the gastric bubble was not made in a scientific way, but as scientifically valuable reports appeared in the medical literature, confirmation was obtained that the method was not an effective method of weight control and that it produced too many severe side-effects. By 1988, the gastric bubble had been deflated!

The current situation

At present, vertical gastric stapling or banding via a laparoscope are the preferred methods of inducing weight loss, as it seems to be as effective as other methods and has few long-term complications, either physical or psychological.

The patient must clearly understand, before operation, that the creation of a smaller stomach during an operation which may last one to two hours will not cure a lifetime's addiction to food or alter disordered eating habits. The patient must also be aware that, following operation, vitamin and mineral supplements are necessary, pain may occur, as may episodes of diarrhoea, and appropriate follow-up, including blood-tests, is essential. Patients should consider surgery as an adjunct to weight loss and not a substitute for sensible eating and exercise.

Case history: Gareth

I was always pretty big and when I was 16 I played Rugby League. Then I weighed about 89 kg (196 lbs, 14 st; BMI 27), but it was all muscle—no fat. That's when I started working in the blast furnace. I drank like a fish and ate like a horse but worked it out and sweated it out so I didn't put on any weight in that job. I didn't like the job much and so I got this job with the railways. The problem was that in the new job I just sat down for 8–10 hours a day and mostly did nothing, but I still had the same eating and drinking habits. So I started putting on weight and got up to 153 kg (337 lbs, 24 st 1 lb; BMI 46). I was so fat I found it hard to do my job. The railway doctor said I'd have to lose weight or he'd take me off driving. I tried diets, Weight Watchers, and all the rest, but it didn't do any good. When you work shifts there's no way you can keep to a diet. I drank a lot of coffee and when you have coffee you have to have biscuits or a sandwich. Then I tried exercise. That didn't work either. I'd play football and then go to the pub. Playing made me hungry. So I ate more.

About this time I read about some operations and experiments they were doing in the States. Someone was telling me about it where they put a plastic tube inside your intestines so that the wall couldn't absorb the food as it was blocked off. So I went and saw my doctor about it and straight out he said 'I don't agree with it. You are overweight but you have a big frame. You are a big boned boy and you can carry that weight with no trouble. As far as I am concerned, if you can't lose weight on a diet you're going to have to put up with it'. Then I was over at another doctor and she started asking me about my weight. I told her I had asked my doctor about it and she said 'Oh, go and see this bloke' and sent me off to my surgeon.

He told me about the two types of operations he was doing at the time, one that he was doing before where he stitched across the stomach and took a piece of the bowel out and rerouted it into the top of the stomach. He also told me about his other one that he eventually did on me. And that was to make my stomach smaller by stapling across it. He called it gastric partitioning.

He did the operation one Wednesday. I didn't feel too bad after it, I was doped up to my ears the first couple of days with pain-killers and

Case history: Gareth (continued)

felt nothing. Bill—that's my surgeon—is one of these blokes who are sticklers for exercise and I was up walking around the second day though the walk was more like a slow crawl. He told me I wouldn't want to eat much because I would feel full quickly. When I was in hospital and did start eating again it was on a puree diet, everything blended and only in very small amounts. When I came home I stayed on the puree for a while then gradually started experimenting around with what I could take and what I couldn't. Before I had the operation I would eat a 2 lb rump steak and have a couple of beers and a bottle of wine. But I couldn't do that after the operation. I felt full quickly and if I didn't chew the food into small pieces, up it would come. It couldn't get through the hole or something. Bill had told me that before the operation. He told me what I would be able to eat but that everything would have to be chewed thoroughly until it was pulp because it had to go through the hole of about 1/8 or 1/4 of an inch. If you don't chew it enough to let it go through there it comes back. So I adjusted my eating habits. I ate less and chewed well. I still get some regurgitation but not much. I think I'm a hell of a lot fitter than I was before and I think that because I carried the weight for so long I'm a lot fitter than many other blokes. For example, I suppose about 12 months after the operation I went along to the beach to do a bit of jogging to see how far I could go. I used to be able to jog a mile, no worries, when I was overweight. Well, I went from one end of the beach to the other and back and three-quarters of the way back again, which would probably be nearer 4 or 5 miles and I wasn't even puffing at the end of it, no strain, no nothing, just felt like a walk across the road.

The operation made me change how much I ate and how I ate. It also stopped me drinking beer. Wine is OK, but the gas in beer blows your stomach up and it hurts.

I had a problem about two years after the operation. It seemed the hole had got narrower and I couldn't keep anything down—even water. So I saw Bill, and he said 'Back to hospital, over you go'. They put a gastric tube down and pumped my stomach out, put a drip in to feed me and I stayed there for 3 days. They put a thing down to have a look, couldn't see anything and Bill said 'We'll have to open you up and find out what is wrong'. So he opened it up, fixed it and found I had a few gallstones so he took the gallbladder while he was there, and since that I've been well. I'm down to 70 kg (154 lbs, 11 st; BMI 22). I can go out and eat a meal. I don't eat much red meat and I'm off steaks because by the time you've cut it up small and chewed it, the rest is cold. I'm

> *Case history: Gareth* (continued)
> life. But it is good to know that I can contact Bill if anything goes
> wrong.
>   Would I have had the operation if I'd known what it meant?
> Thinking back I would, but when I came out of surgery and for a couple
> of weeks after that and the two lots of surgery I've had, up until 6
> months ago, I doubted whether I would. One of the blokes at work has
> just been recommended to have it done and he asked me if I would
> recommend it. I said 'No, I wouldn't recommend it, but if you want it,
> have it, it helped me.'

Table 42. The appropriate management of morbid obesity

Appropriate	Inappropriate
Low energy, nutritionally balanced menu plan for more than 6 months	Complex crazy fat diets
	Excessive exercise with dieting
Moderate regular exercise	Sauna baths
Cognitive behaviour therapy	Electric treatment
Supportive psychotherapy, and help from a dietitian	
? Anorectic drugs	Diuretics
(short-term: less than 4 months)	Thyroid hormones
If failure:	
Surgery	
? Jaw-wiring	Jejuno-ileal bypass
Gastric reduction lap banding	Gastric balloon (bubble)

Diane asked me to give to readers some advice about lap-bands.
'*Tell people lap-bands are only aids to losing weight . . . they do not do the
job . . . you can still eat a lot with a lap-band but not too much solid food
. . . you can undermine it by melting chocolate in the microwave or living
on milkshakes, it does work but you have to be committed.*'

Diane age 55 years was brought up in a family with an abundance
of food and feelings of being loved by her parents. As a child her
father was often hungry and promised his family they would always
have enough to eat. Food was bought in bulk, never as single
items. There were five well-stocked refrigerators in the home.
Both her parents drank excessive amounts of alcohol and were

seldom at home. Her father, who became jealous and violent when he had been drinking, drank at the local pub while her mother frequented the more up-market clubs. Diane was the eldest of 7 children and was responsible for bringing up the first six. She was expected to go straight home from school every day to look after them. She left home when her mother became pregnant with the seventh child.

Diane describes herself as 'chubby as a baby and always overweight' and felt that being overweight at school 'was the least of my problems'. At school she was teased for being dirty and 'smelling bad' and asked to sit away from the other children in the classroom. She had only one school uniform and one dress to wear to church each Sunday. The house was always chaotic, untidy, and dirty, and clothes washing was only done episodically. In many ways the children were neglected. Other families in her area considered her family undesirable.

As she was growing up sometimes Diane liked being overweight and acting 'rough' to annoy her mother who dressed well, was slim, and acted in a ladylike manner. To escape from home at 19 years she asked for a transfer of her job to interstate. Once interstate she enjoyed her life and was popular with friends and had boyfriends until she married at age 30. She lost weight during a holiday age 19 years and reached what she felt was a normal weight and felt she looked lovely (about 90 kg) (200 lbs; BMI 28). At work she is very conscientious and works until she has finishes each job. She has always been in great demand and very successful as a private secretary; she had travelled overseas, saved, and bought her own home before she married. Over the years her weight gradually increased to 126 kg (20 stone, 280 lbs; BMI 41) at age 33 when she became pregnant with her first child. She felt she had tried every popular diet recommended by magazines and doctors, acupuncture, multiple medications prescribed by doctors, participated in clubs and weight loss groups on many occasions, and attended exercise groups and gyms. 'When I was pregnant I gave up smoking and (although she seldom drank alcohol) stopped drinking. I am a very disciplined person, why can't I stop myself eating?' In the year following the birth of her son she was 155 kg (23 stone, 322 lbs; BMI 50). She failed to become pregnant again and sought help for her infertility. In desperation she agreed to an operation to reduce the length of her small intestine. A weight loss of 50 kg (98 lbs) occurred in the following 12 to 18 months. She became pregnant spontaneously and was delighted by the birth of a healthy baby daughter. Two years after her surgery her weight gradually began to increase back to her present weight. 'It was 20 years of chronic diarrhoea, wind pain . . . I hated going to the toilet the pain was so bad, the smell was awful and I had bacterial infections so had to take tablets. I had it reversed six months ago and had a lap-band inserted.

'I've been successful at everything I have set out to do except lose weight. When I have problems I always think I deserve something, the only thing I want is food. Recently a dietitian asked me to list things I find comforting. I could not think of anything except food, it is my comfort and my reward.' Diane buys in bulk and hoards food. She fears feeling hungry and always has food with her. Nowadays she will take two pieces of fruit with her if she is driving somewhere, one piece for the outward trip and one piece for the trip home. Previously this would have been two bags of sweets. To stop herself buying food, especially cakes, she has given large amounts of money to people collecting for charities in shopping centres. Binge-eating is very rare and the two occasions of feeling urgently compelled to get food and eat were related to external stressful events. It is possible Diane would binge-eat more often if she did not always keep food with her.

Until the last two years when she started to develop knee problems because of the excess weight, Diane considered the worst feature of being overweight was embarrassing her children. A child at preschool asked her daughter if her mother was pregnant or just fat. Although she always dressed well she felt she should not attend her children's school functions, as her children might be humiliated. The rest of the time she felt she successfully maintained the myth of the fat and happy girl who was fun loving and joined in everything. She felt good about herself when she could do things for others and please them. Although it is early days the lap-band is improving her self-esteem. She knows she is losing weight and she is attending a weight control clinic (included as part of the surgery) each week. She is following what she has been advised and is being encouraged to do this by her clinic dietitians and surgeon. Not to drink before, during, or 30 minutes after meals as the food can swell up and get stuck, and not to drink anything cold before eating as it can make the stoma (hole) smaller which makes it difficult to eat. The other advice is to exercise.

'I can now walk the whole length of the shopping centre without sitting down and I can swim over 600 metres (700 yards) in 30 minutes. I wish I could bottle up the good feeling I have when I have exercised and eaten well, if only I could feel this when I am tempted to eat too much yogurt.'

Suction lipectomy (liposuction)

Rather than being generally obese, some individuals tend to deposit fat on their hips and thighs. This is probably an inherited characteristic. There is a belief that the fat cells (adipocytes) in these areas multiply when faced with the need to store fat, whilst the adipocytes of the abdomen, the back, and the upper arms tend to expand considerably before they multiply. The appearance of the thighs has given rise to the name of 'cellulite'.

Suction lipectomy, which is a method of removing localized fat deposits, has been used to remove fat from below the chin, from the sides of the chest, from the fat over the lower abdomen, the hips, and the thighs.

The technique is simple but problems may occur. A small incision is made in the skin over the area and a hollow tube, called a cannula, is introduced through this incision to make radiating tunnels in the fatty tissues under the skin. The fatty tissue is sucked through the cannula. Following the surgery, a compression bandage has to be wrapped firmly around the area for about ten days, and support garments have to be worn for a further six weeks.

Many people suffer from bruising under the skin after suction lipectomy, and often the area becomes swollen. This leads to an uneven skin which may last for two or three months. Most people feel pain and discomfort following suction lipectomy.

Suction lipectomy is not a treatment for generalized obesity, but it may be useful to remove unsightly fatty deposits, particularly in people of normal weight. The best results occur if an experienced surgeon performs the procedure.

The physical and psychological benefits of weight reduction in gross obesity

In spite of the dangers of operations for gross obesity, in spite of complications which may follow surgery, in spite of the need for careful

Table 43. Summary of treatment strategies for obesity

Mild or moderate obesity
- remember that obesity is determined by genetic as well as environmental factors
- choose a menu plan which reduces your energy intake considerably
- remember that weight loss is a slow process, there is no miracle diet and exercise
- long-term weight management is about enjoyable, realistic eating and exercise
- to succeed, you have to be motivated to lose weight
- cognitive-behaviour therapy can help binge-eating

Severe or (morbid) obesity
If the measures for treating mild or moderate obesity fail, consider (with your doctor) the following:
- seeking help, counselling, or cognitive-behaviour therapy from an obesity specialist and a dietitian. They may suggest that you:
- choose a very low calorie diet
- try one of the newer antiobesity medications

If the above fail, or after trying them you regain the lost weight, consider gastric reduction in conjunction with sensible eating and exercise

---

attention to diet, in spite of the need for vitamin and mineral supplements, and the need for frequent visits for 'follow-up', the choice must ultimately be that of the patient. There is no doubt of the physical benefits of weight reduction. Cardiac function improves and the level of the blood pressure is reduced, which reduces the risk of a stroke. The blood circulation to the legs improves with reduction in thrombophlebitis. There is an improvement in pulmonary ventilation, with a reduction in shortness of breath. If the person has osteoarthritis, or low back pain, the severity of the pain is reduced. Following a significant reduction in weight there is an increase in energy and a reduction in fatigue.

The psychological benefits of surgical measures to achieve weight reduction have been less clearly delineated. As weight loss progresses, patients perceive their bodies more favourably and become more self-confident about their personality. The majority of women see themselves as more feminine and more sexually attractive; however, there is no change in the frequency of sexual activity or in sexual pleasure. They experience fewer mood changes and see themselves as more self-assured, outgoing, and comfortable. They become more sociable, less preoccupied by weight, and less likely to eat more than they intended at meals or between meals. In spite of these positive findings, many others still feel that they are large, and in psychological tests tend to over-estimate their body size.

These findings suggest that grossly obese people who have failed to reduce their weight significantly by dieting, or fail to maintain the lower weight, may benefit physically and psychologically from surgery, but must weigh up the advantages and disadvantages of the operations.

Appendix a: Body Mass Index (BMI) charts

BMI CHARTS

Height	Height	Height²	BMI 17	BMI 18	BMI 19	BMI 20	BMI 25	BMI 30	BMI 35	BMI 40
[Ft.in]	[m]	[m²]	[kg]	[kg]	[kg]	[kg]	[kg]	[kg]	[kg]	[kg]
	1.45	2.10	35.70	37.80	40.00	42.00	52.50	63.00	73.50	84.00
	1.46	2.13	36.20	38.30	40.50	42.60	53.30	63.90	74.60	85.00
4–10	1.47	2.16	36.70	38.80	41.00	43.20	54.00	64.80	75.60	86.00
	1.48	2.19	37.20	39.40	41.60	43.80	54.80	65.70	76.70	88.00
	1.49	2.22	37.70	40.00	42.20	44.40	55.50	66.60	77.70	89.00
4–11	1.50	2.25	38.30	40.50	42.80	45.00	56.30	67.50	78.80	90.00
	1.51	2.28	38.80	41.00	43.30	45.60	57.00	68.40	79.80	91.00
5–0	1.52	2.31	39.30	41.60	43.90	46.20	57.80	69.30	80.90	92.00
	1.53	2.34	39.80	42.10	44.50	46.80	58.50	70.20	81.90	94.00
	1.54	2.37	40.30	42.70	45.10	47.40	59.30	71.10	83.00	95.00

BMI CHARTS (continued)

Height [ft.in]	Height [m]	Height [m2]	BMI 17 [kg]	BMI 18 [kg]	BMI 19 [kg]	BMI 20 [kg]	BMI 25 [kg]	BMI 30 [kg]	BMI 35 [kg]	BMI 40 [kg]
5-1	1.55	2.40	40.80	43.20	45.70	48.00	60.00	72.00	84.00	96.00
	1.56	2.43	41.30	43.70	46.20	48.60	60.80	72.90	85.10	97.00
	1.57	2.47	42.00	44.50	46.80	49.40	61.80	74.10	86.50	99.00
5-2	1.58	2.50	42.50	45.00	47.40	50.00	62.50	75.00	87.50	100.00
	1.59	2.53	43.00	45.50	48.00	50.60	63.25	75.90	88.60	101.00
5-3	1.60	2.56	43.50	46.10	48.60	51.20	64.00	76.80	89.60	102.00
	1.61	2.59	44.00	46.60	49.20	51.80	64.80	77.70	90.70	103.00
	1.62	2.62	44.50	47.20	49.90	52.40	65.50	78.60	91.70	105.00
5-4	1.63	2.66	45.20	47.90	50.50	53.20	66.50	79.80	93.10	106.00
	1.64	2.69	45.70	48.40	51.10	53.80	67.30	80.70	94.20	108.00
5-5	1.65	2.72	46.20	49.00	51.70	54.40	68.00	81.70	95.20	109.00
	1.66	2.76	46.90	49.70	52.40	55.20	69.00	82.80	96.60	110.00
	1.67	2.79	47.40	50.20	53.00	55.80	69.80	83.70	97.70	112.00
5-6	1.68	2.82	47.90	50.80	53.60	56.40	70.50	84.60	98.70	113.00
	1.69	2.86	48.60	51.50	54.30	57.20	71.50	85.80	100.10	114.00
5-7	1.70	2.89	49.10	52.00	54.90	57.80	72.30	86.70	101.20	116.00
	1.71	2.92	49.60	52.60	55.60	58.40	73.00	87.60	102.20	117.00
	1.72	2.96	50.30	53.30	56.20	59.20	74.00	88.80	103.60	118.00
5-8	1.73	2.99	50.80	53.30	56.80	59.80	74.80	89.70	104.70	120.00
	1.74	3.03	51.50	54.50	57.50	60.60	75.80	91.00	106.10	121.00

BMI CHARTS *(continued)*

Height	Height	Height	BMI 17	BMI 18	BMI 19	BMI 20	BMI 25	BMI 30	BMI 35	BMI 40
[ft.in]	[m]	[m2]	[kg]	[kg]	[kg]	[kg]	[kg]	[kg]	[kg]	[kg]
5–9	1.75	3.06	52.00	55.10	58.20	61.20	76.50	91.80	107.10	122.00
	1.76	3.10	52.70	55.80	58.90	62.00	77.50	93.00	108.50	124.00
	1.77	3.13	53.20	56.30	59.50	62.60	78.30	94.00	109.60	125.00
5–10	1.78	3.17	53.90	57.10	60.20	63.40	79.30	95.10	111.00	127.00
	1.79	3.20	54.50	57.60	60.80	64.00	80.00	96.00	112.00	128.00
5–11	1.80	3.24	55.10	58.30	61.60	64.80	81.00	97.20	113.40	130.00
	1.81	3.28	55.76	59.04	62.32	65.60	82.00	98.00	115.00	131.00
	1.82	3.31	56.27	59.58	62.89	66.20	82.75	99.00	116.00	132.00
6–0	1.83	3.35	56.95	60.30	63.65	67.00	83.75	100.50	117.00	134.00
	1.84	3.38	57.46	60.84	64.22	67.60	84.50	101.00	118.00	135.00
	1.85	3.42	58.14	61.56	64.98	68.40	85.50	103.00	120.00	137.00
6–1	1.86	3.46	58.82	62.28	65.74	69.20	86.50	104.00	121.00	138.00
	1.87	3.50	59.50	63.00	66.50	70.00	87.50	105.00	123.00	140.00
6–2	1.88	3.53	60.01	63.54	67.07	70.60	88.25	106.00	124.00	141.00
	1.89	3.57	60.69	64.26	67.83	71.40	89.25	107.00	125.00	142.00
	1.90	3.61	61.37	64.78	68.59	72.20	90.25	108.00	126.00	144.00
6–3	1.91	3.65	62.05	65.71	69.35	73.00	91.25	110.00	128.00	146.00

BMI = weight (kg) ÷ height (m)^2

Appendix b: pounds to kilograms chart

POUNDS TO KILOGRAMS

Pounds	Kg	Pounds	Kg	Pounds	Kg	Pounds	Kg
1 lb	0.45 kg	50 lb	22.7 kg	99 lb	44.9 kg	148 lb	67.0 kg
2 lb	0.91 kg	51 lb	23.1 kg	100 lb	45.3 kg	149 lb	67.4 kg
3 lb	1.36 kg	52 lb	23.6 kg	101 lb	45.7 kg	150 lb	67.9 kg
4 lb	1.81 kg	53 lb	24.0 kg	102 lb	46.2 kg	151 lb	68.4 kg
5 lb	2.27 kg	54 lb	24.5 kg	103 lb	46.7 kg	152 lb	68.8 kg
6 lb	2.72 kg	55 lb	24.9 kg	104 lb	47.1 kg	153 lb	69.2 kg
7 lb	3.18 kg	56 lb (4 st)	25.4 kg	105 lb	47.6 kg	154 lb (11 st)	69.7 kg
8 lb	3.63 kg	57 lb	25.9 kg	106 lb	48.0 kg	155 lb	70.2 kg
9 lb	4.08 kg	58 lb	26.3 kg	107 lb	48.5 kg	156 lb	70.6 kg
10 lb	4.54 kg	59 lb	26.8 kg	108 lb	49.0 kg	157 lb	71.0 kg
11 lb	4.99 kg	60 lb	27.2 kg	109 lb	49.4 kg	158 lb	71.5 kg
12 lb	5.44 kg	61 lb	27.7 kg	110 lb	49.8 kg	159 lb	71.9 kg
13 lb	5.90 kg	62 lb	28.1 kg	111 lb	50.3 kg	160 lb	72.4 kg
14 lb (1 st)	6.35 kg	63 lb	28.6 kg	112 lb (8 st)	50.8 kg	161 lb	72.8 kg
15 lb	6.80 kg	64 lb	29.0 kg	113 lb	51.2 kg	162 lb	73.3 kg
16 lb	7.26 kg	65 lb	29.5 kg	114 lb	51.7 kg	163 lb	73.7 kg
17 lb	7.71 kg	66 lb	29.9 kg	115 lb	52.1 kg	164 lb	74.2 kg
18 lb	8.16 kg	67 lb	30.4 kg	116 lb	52.6 kg	165 lb	74.6 kg
19 lb	8.62 kg	68 lb	30.8 kg	117 lb	53.0 kg	166 lb	75.1 kg
20 lb	9.07 kg	69 lb	31.3 kg	118 lb	53.5 kg	167 lb	75.5 kg
21 lb	9.52 kg	70 lb (5 st)	31.7 kg	119 lb	53.9 kg	168 lb (12 st)	76.0 kg
22 lb	9.98 kg	71 lb	32.1 kg	120 lb	54.4 kg	169 lb	76.4 kg
23 lb	10.43 kg	72 lb	32.6 kg	121 lb	54.9 kg	170 lb	76.9 kg
24 lb	10.89 kg	73 lb	33.0 kg	122 lb	55.3 kg	171 lb	77.4 kf
25 lb	11.34 kg	74 lb	33.5 kg	123 lb	55.7 kg	172 lb	77.8 kg
26 lb	11.79 kg	75 lb	34.0 kg	124 lb	56.2 kg	173 lb	78.3 kg
27 lb	12.25 kg	76 lb	34.4 kg	125 lb	56.5 kg	174 lb	78.7 kg
28 lb (2 st)	12.70 kg	77 lb	34.8 kg	126 lb (9 st)	57.1 kg	175 lb	79.2 kg

POUNDS TO KILOGRAMS (continued)

Pounds	Kg	Pounds	Kg	Pounds	Kg	Pounds	Kg
29 lb	13.2 kg	78 lb	35.3 kg	127 lb	57.5 kg	176 lb	79.6 kg
30 lb	13.6 kg	79 lb	35.8 kg	128 lb	58.0 kg	177 lb	80.0 kg
31 lb	14.1 kg	80 lb	36.3 kg	129 lb	58.4 kg	178 lb	80.5 kg
32 lb	14.5 kg	81 lb	36.7 kg	130 lb	58.9 kg	179 lb	80.9 kg
33 lb	15.0 kg	82 lb	37.3 kg	131 lb	59.3 kg	180 lb	81.4 kg
34 lb	15.4 kg	83 lb	37.6 kg	132 lb	59.8 kg	181 lb	81.8 kg
35 lb	15.9 kg	84 lb (6 st)	38.1 kg	133 lb	60.2 kg	182 lb (13 st)	82.3 kg
36 lb	16.3 kg	85 lb	38.5 kg	134 lb	60.7 kg	183 lb	82.7 kg
37 lb	16.8 kg	86 lb	39.0 kg	135 lb	61.1 kg	184 lb	83.2 kg
38 lb	17.2 kg	87 lb	39.4 kg	136 lb	61.6 kg	185 lb	83.6 kg
39 lb	17.7 kg	88 lb	39.9 kg	137 lb	62.1 kg	186 lb	84.1 kg
40 lb	18.1 kg	89 lb	40.3 kg	138 lb	62.5 kg	187 lb	84.5 kg
41 lb	18.6 kg	90 lb	40.8 kg	139 lb	62.9 kg	188 lb	85.0 kg
42 lb (3 st)	19.0 kg	91 lb	41.2 kg	140 lb (10 st)	63.4 kg	189 lb	85.5 kg
43 lb	19.5 kg	92 lb	41.7 kg	141 lb	63.8 kg	190 lb	85.9 kg
44 lb	20.0 kg	93 lb	42.2 kg	142 lb	64.3 kg	191 lb	86.3 kg
45 lb	20.4 kg	94 lb	42.6 kg	143 lb	64.7 kg	192 lb	86.8 kg
46 lb	20.9 kg	95 lb	43.0 kg	144 lb	65.2 kg	193 lb	87.3 kg
47 lb	21.3 kg	96 lb	43.5 kg	145 lb	65.6 kg	194 lb	87.7 kg
48 lb	21.8 kg	97 lb	44.0 kg	146 lb	66.1 kg	195 lb	88.2 kg
49 lb	22.2 kg	98 lb (7 st)	44.5 kg	147 lb	66.5 kg	196 lb (14 st)	88.6 kg

Further reading

Abraham, S. and Lovell, N. *Eating and exercise examination by computer* (EEE-C). (1999).

This manual describes the assessment of eating disorders and the criteria used. This is the first fully computerized assessment, analysis, and reporting instrument to be developed.

Brownell, K.D. and Fairburn, C. *A comprehensive textbook of eating disorders and obesity.* Guildford Publications, New York (1995).

This textbook covers and integrates information about eating disorders and obesity. It consists of articles from over 100 leading international experts in the field and provides an up-to-date review of the state of regulation of eating and weight, body image, diagnosis, assessment, treatment, and prognosis of eating disorders. It is a valuable reference book, if somewhat biased towards American authors.

Bruch, Hilda. *Eating disorders, obesity, anorexia nervosa and the person within.* Routledge Kegan Paul, London (1974) and *The golden cage.* Open Books, Somerset (1978).

Before writing this book Hilda Bruch had been involved in treatment of people with eating disorders for 40 years. She believes that people develop an eating disorder to avoid having to cope with an aspect of their life. She stresses that treatment must be individual and that the aim is not only to restore normal eating behaviour but to ensure the happiness of the 'person within'.

Cooper, P. *Bulimia nervosa and binge-eating—a guide to recovery.* Robinson, London (1995).

This short book contains a self-help manual, based on the cognitive-behavioural approach to treatment. It may appeal to eating disorder sufferers who are reluctant to seek professional help.

Crisp, A. *Anorexia nervosa—Let me be.* Academic Press, London (1980).

Crisp's theory is that young women develop anorexia nervosa because they seek to return to being a child biologically and, in many ways, socially and psychologically. They fear the challenges of adolescence, with its maturative and sexual connotations.

Dally, P. and Gomez, J. *Obesity and anorexia nervosa—A question of shape.* Faber, London (1990).

This book gives an outline of the problem of eating disorders, and describes the ways in which treatment is undertaken. Written for the general reader it gives much information in a clear, concise way.

Fairburn, Christopher. *Overcoming binge-eating.* Guildford Press, New York (1995).

A self-help manual, similar to Peter Cooper's book. Recommended.

Fairburn, C.G. and Wilson, G.T. (eds). *Binge-eating: nature, assessment, and treatment.* Guildford Press, New York (1995).

A book for health professionals written by 19 experts, which covers much of the published material about bulimia nervosa. One of the book's strengths is that it has a chapter with a detailed discussion on cognitive-behavioural therapy and a practical description of the eating disorders examination (EDE).

Garfinkle, P.E. and Garner, D.M. *Anorexia nervosa, a multidimensional perspective.* Brunner Mazel, New York (1983).

Although old, this is an excellent book, written for health professionals. The extensive literature about anorexia nervosa, and anorexia nervosa with bulimia nervosa episodes, is critically evaluated. The many studies made by the Toronto group are reported and placed in perspective. The book is written in lucid English and integrates the physiological, psychological, and clinical aspects of a complex, multi-dimensional eating disorder.

Garner, D. and Garfinkle, P. *Handbook of treatment for eating disorders.* 2nd edition, Guildford press, New York (1997).

This is one of the more recent reference books by well-known authors and specialists in eating disorders.

Garrow, J.S. *Treat obesity seriously.* Churchill-Livingstone, Edinburgh (1988).

Dr Garrow has headed a research group into nutritional problems for some years and has written extensively about obesity. This book is designed to help general practitioners and general (fat?) readers understand the biological problems associated with obesity. A personal account, it gives an excellent review of the problems and of treatment strategies.

Palmer, R.L. *Anorexia nervosa—A guide for sufferers and their families*. Penguin, Harmondsworth (1989).

Trained at St. George's Medical School, Palmer supports Crisp's view that anorexia nervosa is due to a psychobiological regression to childhood. Written for the general reader, the book acquaints sufferers from anorexia nervosa and their families of the possibilities for treatment and of the probable outcomes.

Schnidt, U. and Treasure, J. *Getting better bit(e) by bit(e)*. Lawrence Erlbaum Associates (1993).

A self-help manual. Recommended.

Glossary

Adipose tissue The tissues of the body which contain numbers of fat cells. Adipose tissue is 80 per cent fat, 2 per cent protein, and 18 per cent water. Because of the large proportion of fat, adipose tissue is often called fatty tissue.

Alkalosis An increase in the alkalinity of the blood, which normally is slightly acidic. It is usually due to an increase in the level of bicarbonate in the blood.

Amenorrhoea The cessation or absence of menstruation for more than 3 months.

Anastomose To join together two hollow tubes; in this case to join the stomach to the intestine.

Anorexia nervosa See p. 26 for diagnostic criteria.

Anovulation Lack of ovulation over a period of months.

Average Body Weight (ABW) The average body weight for age, height, and weight.

Bariatric physician A doctor who specializes in treating obesity.

Behaviour therapy A psychological therapy based on experimental psychology, intended to change symptoms and behaviour by various techniques, for example, anxiety management training, assertiveness training, aversion therapy, biofeedback, and desensitization.

Biceps The muscle extending from the shoulder to the elbow joint, on the front surface of the arm.

Body Mass Index (BMI) A measure devised over 100 years ago to determine whether a person is of normal weight, underweight, or obese. The calculation is made in the following way:

$$\frac{\text{Weight in kilograms}}{\text{Height in metres} \times \text{Height in metres}}$$

For example, a woman aged 24 weighs 46 kg and is 1.57 metres tall:

$$46 \div 1.57 \times 1.57 = 18.6$$

The index of 18.6 indicates that she is underweight.

Bulimia nervosa See p. 32 for definition.

Calories A lay term for kilocalories (see entry for kilocalories).

Carbohydrates The class of nutrients made up of starches and sugars. Carbohydrates provide the main source of energy needed for the human body to function. Starches are the most common form of dietary carbohydrate, and are found in cereal grains, roots, and tubers. In the human gut starches are broken down to sugars, finally to glucose, which is absorbed into the blood.

Chorionic gonadotrophin A hormone derived from the placenta which was used to treat obesity. Also known as human chorionic gonadotrophin, or HCG.

Cognitive-behavioural therapy Psychological therapy intended to change maladaptive ways of thinking and thereby bring about improvement in psychological disorders. In other words, a technique used to help people think differently so that they will behave differently.

Diuretics Drugs which act on the kidney to increase the flow of urine.

Electrolyte A substance which, dissolved in water, separates into electrically charged particles (ions) capable of conducting an electrical current.

Flatus 'Wind' or gas accumulated in the bowel and expelled through the anus (back passage).

Follicle-stimulating hormone (FSH) A hormone secreted by the pituitary gland that stimulates the growth of the egg follicles in the ovary and the development of sperm in the testis.

Gastroplasty An operation on the stomach in which a small section is 'partitioned', so that the size of the stomach is effectively reduced.

Glycogen The form in which sugars and starches are stored in animals. Sucrose and starches from plants are converted into glucose before being absorbed into the human body from the gut, and the glucose is converted into glycogen for storage in the liver and in muscle.

Gonadotrophin A substance, usually a hormone, capable of stimulating the ovaries or the testicles (trophin means growth).

Gonadotrophic releasing hormone (GnRH) A substance secreted by the hypothalamus which is carried by blood vessels to the pituitary gland to stimulate the production and release of the gonadotrophic hormones.

Haematemesis Bloody vomit.

Hypertension High blood pressure.

Hypothalamus The part of the brain just above the brain-stem which controls the activity of the pituitary gland.

Ketosis An accumulation of excessive amounts of chemical compounds in the tissues, which produces acidity in the body tissues and fluids.

Kilocalorie A kilocalorie (also called Kcalories, Kcals, or calories) is a measure of the energy in foods. It is defined as the amount of heat required to raise the temperature of a litre of water from 15°C to 16°C. Each food contains a different amount of energy, which is absorbed into the body after eating and expended to keep the body functioning. Recently kcals have been replaced by a new energy measurement called a kilojoule 1 kcal = 4.19 kJ.

Kilojoule Measure of energy, which has replaced the kilocalorie. One kilojoule = 0.24 kilocalories.

Lanugo Soft, downy hair, similar to that found in small babies.

Laxatives Drugs which act on the bowel to increase the speed of the passage of food and of the stools through the gut. They cause soft and frequent motions.

Libido A person's sexual desire, arousal, and awareness.

Luteinizing hormone (LH) A hormone secreted by and released from the pituitary gland which leads to the release of a mature egg (or ovum) from an ovarian follicle and converts the follicle into a corpus luteum (or yellow body).

Megajoule This is a measure of energy in foods, or expended by the body. 1 megajoule (MJ) = 1000 kilojoule (kJ) = 239 kcals.

Menarche The onset of menstruation.

Millilitre (ml) Equivalent to 0.035 fluid ounces.

Obesity See p. 238 for definition.

Osteomalacia Thinning of the bones.

Peristalsis The wave-like, progressive, sequential movement of the wall of the intestines which churns up food and moves it on towards the anus.

Picking behaviour Moving from food in cupboard, to pantry, to fridge, to pick and eat small quantities of various foods.

Pituitary gland The gland located at the base of the brain that affects the function of other glands by releasing special hormones.

Placebo A harmless substance administered to test the effectiveness of an active substance in a scientific study.

Quetelet Index See Body Mass Index.

Resistance behaviour Behaviour used as methods of stopping abnormal eating patterns.

Resting metabolic rate The resting metabolic rate can be calculated from the formula:

$$RMR = 99.8 \ (\text{body weight in kg} \times 1.155) + (\text{total body potassium} \times 0.0223) - (\text{age} \times 0.456).$$

The result is expressed as the oxygen uptake in ml/minute. If this figure is multiplied by 7, a rough approximation of the energy expenditure (in kilocals) is obtained.

Satiety (Satiation) The feeling of 'fullness' after eating food.

Steatorrhoea Offensive, loose, 'fatty' stools.

Suprailiac The region of the body just above the pelvic bones which identifies a person's waist.

Triceps The muscle on the back of the upper arm.

Venous thrombosis A clot in a vein.

Index